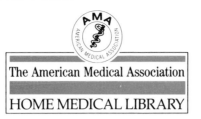

The American Medical Association

HOME MEDICAL LIBRARY

DIAGNOSING DISEASE

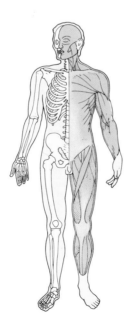

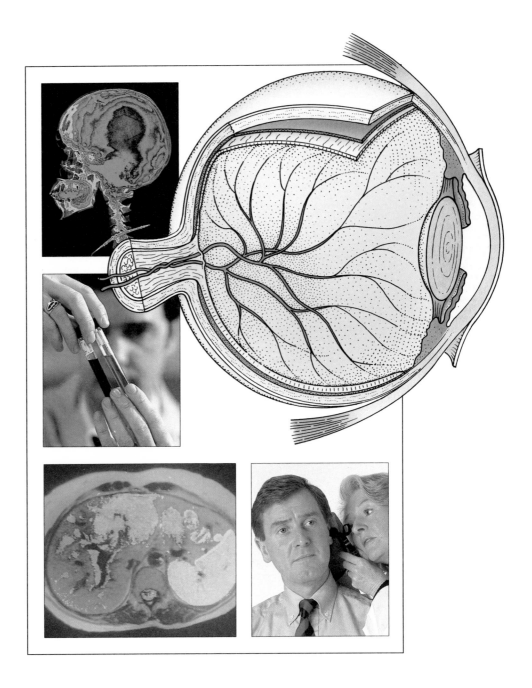

THE AMERICAN
MEDICAL ASSOCIATION

DIAGNOSING
DISEASE

Medical Editor
CHARLES B. CLAYMAN, MD

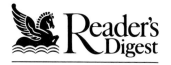

THE READER'S DIGEST ASSOCIATION, INC.
Pleasantville, New York/Montreal

The information in this book reflects current medical knowledge. The
recommendations and information are appropriate in most cases;
however, they are not a substitute for medical diagnosis. For specific
information concerning your personal medical condition, the AMA
suggests that you consult a physician.

The names of organizations, products, or alternative therapies appearing
in this book are given for informational purposes only. Their inclusion
does not imply AMA endorsement, nor does the omission of any
organization, product, or alternative therapy indicate AMA disapproval.

The AMA Home Medical Library is distinct from and unrelated to the series
of health books published by Random House, Inc., in conjunction with the
American Medical Association under the names "The AMA Home
Reference Library" and "The AMA Home Health Library."

Library of Congress Cataloging in Publication Data

American Medical Association.
    Diagnosing disease/the American Medical Association;
medical editor, Charles B. Clayman.
        p. cm. — (The American Medical Association home
medical library)
    Includes index.
    ISBN 0-89577-341-4
    1. Diagnosis — Popular works. I. Clayman, Charles B.
II. Title. III. Series: American Medical Association.
AMA home medical library.
RC71.A54   1989
616.07'5 — dc20   89-10553
                                                          CIP

FOREWORD

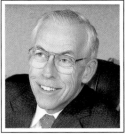

The world is full of people who want to tell you what's wrong if you feel sick. Friends, relatives, and a multitude of self-styled healers may say that they can solve your problems. In what way are medical doctors different from these other sources of advice on health?

This volume of the AMA Home Medical Library explains how and why scientific medicine has a different basis than most other approaches to illness. A medical diagnosis goes beyond treating symptoms; it looks for the underlying cause – the infecting microorganism, the immune system disorder, or a degeneration associated with aging.

Most of us think of scientific medicine as a high-technology pursuit set in the laboratory. However, as the first two chapters in this volume explain, the experienced doctor still spends a long time listening to the patient describe in his or her own words the nature of the illness. This taking of the medical history often points the doctor toward the diagnosis – especially if he or she is an experienced clinician who can compare the current problem with similar consultations.

In many cases, your doctor will have a strong suspicion of what is wrong at the end of the consultation but will want to obtain some clear-cut evidence – if possible – to clinch the diagnosis. You may feel some trepidation or mystification if you are asked to have an X-ray, scan, or an endoscopic examination or if a sample of your blood or tissue is taken for analysis. The later chapters in this volume describe the scientific basis of the range of diagnostic tests in use today, explaining exactly what is done and what the results can show.

We at the American Medical Association hope that the information in this volume will help you feel more at ease – because you will know what to expect – the next time you enter your doctor's office or need to go to the hospital for tests.

JAMES S. TODD, MD
Executive Vice President
American Medical Association

CONTENTS

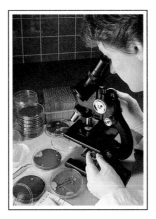

CHAPTER ONE

HOW DISEASES ARE DIAGNOSED

INTRODUCTION

THE DIAGNOSTIC PROCESS

INVESTIGATING THE BODY SYSTEMS

A DOCTOR'S DIAGNOSIS, which precedes treatment, differs in several important ways from the advice given by folk healers or others who are sources of traditional medical care. The folk healer provides a remedy for a symptom (such as headache or constipation) without asking for much more information. By contrast, the key element in a medical diagnosis is the matching of your symptoms and signs to an underlying process produced by disease or altered body function.

Doctors identify diseases by the primary cause. For example, one kind of diarrhea results from bacillary dysentery, an infection of the intestines that is caused by a bacterium. Another type of diarrhea is caused by Crohn's disease, an inflammation of the intestines that is not associated with any known infection. A medical diagnosis requires the elucidation of the primary cause. Thus, "diarrhea" is not a diagnosis, but "bacillary dysentery" or "Crohn's disease" may be. In a similar way, a disorder of the heart, the thyroid gland, the gallbladder, or any other body organ is first classified medically by its cause and by the physical changes it produces.

Knowing the exact cause of a symptom allows the doctor to match it to the past experiences of patients who have the same

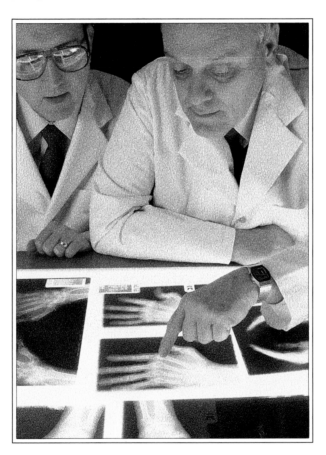

disorder. The doctor can then offer a prognosis, which is a forecast that is based on experience, of the way your illness will develop, how long it will last, and what the final outcome is likely to be. He or she will then be able to say whether a cure is possible or whether therapy can be directed only toward relieving the symptoms or slowing the progress of the disease. To continue the example of diarrhea: if the diagnosis is bacillary dysentery, the doctor can say that it will clear up within a few days if it is treated with fluid replacement and possibly an antibiotic drug. But, if the cause of the diarrhea is Crohn's disease, it is likely to require long-term treatment with anti-inflammatory medications.

This chapter gives an overview of how the doctor reaches a medical diagnosis from the history of the problem, from his or her examination, or from the results of special tests. The first section, THE DIAGNOSTIC PROCESS, describes the overall procedure, from the moment you enter your doctor's office to the point at which he or she reaches the final diagnosis. The second section, INVESTIGATING THE BODY SYSTEMS, reviews the principal methods by which disorders of particular body systems – such as the digestive and nervous systems – are investigated and diagnosed.

9

THE DIAGNOSTIC PROCESS

Pattern recognition
What do diagnosing disease and searching for a face in a crowd have in common? The answer is pattern recognition. Examine, for example, the silhouette of a head, below, then look for the owner of that head in the crowd scene. Using the clues from the silhouette – overall head shape, hairstyle, ear shape, and so on – you will eventually locate the person whose pattern of features most closely matches the clues.

In the same way, a doctor in search of a diagnosis must first seek out clues about a patient's illness. The doctor then mentally reviews his or her knowledge of various diagnostic probabilities – rejecting some imme-

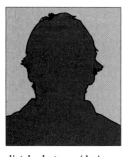

diately, but considering others more carefully – until one is found that most closely accords with the pattern of clues. The diagnosis may come in a sudden flash of realization or may require a lengthy and painstaking search.

Diagnosing disease is essentially a process of pattern recognition. Your doctor recognizes a disease by seeing a pattern formed by your symptoms and by the findings that he or she makes during your physical examination. Laboratory tests can confirm this opinion. The process works in much the same way as recognizing the face of an acquaintance – even after an absence of many years. And, just as some people have a natural ability to remember faces, so, too, a skilled and seasoned doctor has the ability to make a diagnosis on the basis of the patient's appearance and his or her answers to some provocative questions.

Developing an ability for pattern recognition is the basis of medical training. It explains why inexperienced doctors need to spend time accompanying doctors who have years of experience to outpatient clinics or on ward rounds. By integrating this training with his or her knowledge of anatomy and physiology, the inexperienced doctor learns to recognize diseases and disorders. While we learn to recognize our acquaintances mostly by their faces, the doctor looks for clues derived from the physical examination and – most important – from the patient's description of the illness as told in his or her own words.

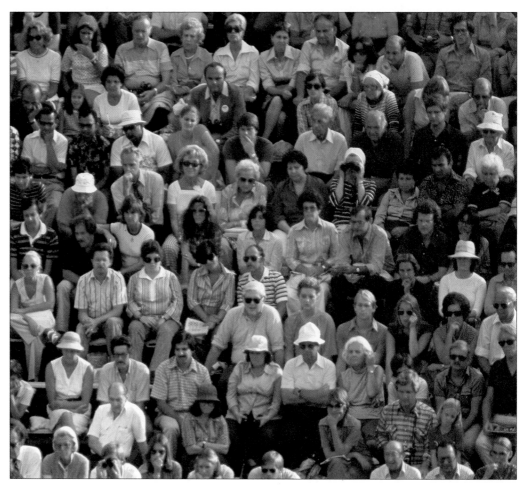

THE CONSULTATION

One of the greatest medical teachers, Sir William Osler, who helped give Johns Hopkins Hospital, Baltimore, Md., its worldwide reputation, said: "Listen to the patient, he is telling you the diagnosis." What Osler meant is that, often, a patient with a certain disorder describes his or her symptoms in words almost identical to those used by others with the same illness. For example, if you tell your doctor that a pain in your stomach wakes you at 2 AM and is relieved when you drink a glass of milk, your doctor will suspect a peptic ulcer because of his or her knowledge of nighttime gastric secretion and because he or she has heard the same description from other patients many times before.

Taking the history

The first stage in diagnosis consists of the doctor listening to the patient describe the main reason for coming to the doctor's office and the details of the illness. The doctor then asks detailed questions based on his or her knowledge of physiology and common patterns of disease. If your description of pain in the chest suggests coronary heart disease, your doctor may ask whether the pain is worse when you walk uphill or whether it is worse in cold weather. The more features your symptoms have in common with the typical description of an illness, the more likely it is that the diagnosis will be correct as deduced from your account.

When the questioning is complete, your doctor will often have a strong suspicion about the most likely cause of your illness. However, he or she will not make a final decision at this point. If your symptoms suggest a disorder of the digestive system, there may be several possibilities that could explain them, ranging from indigestion to stomach cancer. This list of possible disorders is known as the differential diagnosis.

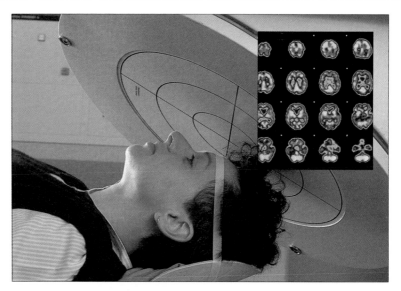

THE PHYSICAL EXAMINATION

After your doctor has made a differential diagnosis, his or her next task is to narrow the list to one or at most two or three possibilities. This is accomplished by performing a physical examination and, in some cases, by ordering special laboratory tests on specimens of your blood and other body fluids. Your doctor may also use X-rays, scans, and other diagnostic procedures.

Medical tests

It is in your best interest that tests be kept to a minimum and cause as little inconvenience as possible. To accomplish this, your doctor initially tests for the first few disorders in his or her differential diagnosis, using the simplest, safest, and least expensive tests. Tests for rarer disorders, using more complex procedures, are usually left until other possibilities have been ruled out.

In recent years, technological advances in laboratory equipment have provided doctors with a far wider range of diagnostic tests. Laboratory techniques are now available for measuring minute quantities of an enormous range of substances in your blood and other body fluids. Imaging techniques have

The imaging revolution
Advances in technology have led to an explosion of diagnostic techniques for imaging the body's organs. The patient above is undergoing brain scanning by a technique called SPECT (single photon emission computed tomography), which provides multiple images of "slices" through the head. Thirty years ago, imaging of the head was largely restricted to plain skull X-rays such as that shown below.

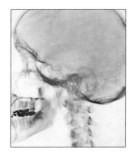

HOW DIAGNOSES ARE REACHED

A diagnosis may be reached at any point during the investigation of a complaint — from the patient's history alone, from the physical examination, or from the doctor's suspicions confirmed by tests. In some cases, the doctor makes a "best guess" at the diagnosis, gives treatment on the basis of this opinion, and determines if the patient's response to treatment confirms or refutes his or her ideas.

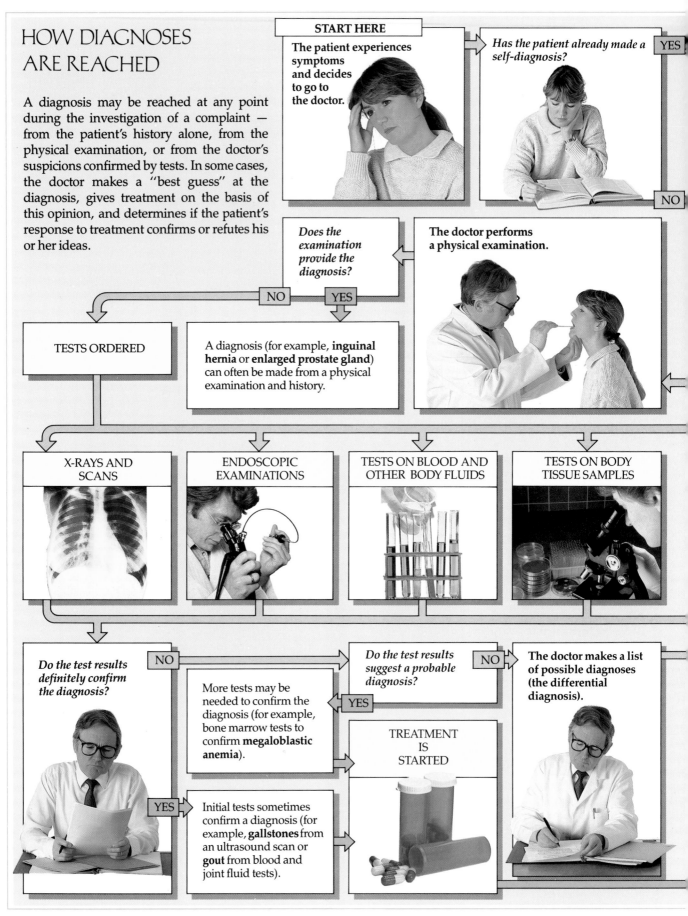

START HERE

The patient experiences symptoms and decides to go to the doctor.

Has the patient already made a self-diagnosis? **YES**

NO

Does the examination provide the diagnosis?

The doctor performs a physical examination.

NO **YES**

TESTS ORDERED

A diagnosis (for example, **inguinal hernia** or **enlarged prostate gland**) can often be made from a physical examination and history.

X-RAYS AND SCANS

ENDOSCOPIC EXAMINATIONS

TESTS ON BLOOD AND OTHER BODY FLUIDS

TESTS ON BODY TISSUE SAMPLES

Do the test results definitely confirm the diagnosis?

NO

More tests may be needed to confirm the diagnosis (for example, bone marrow tests to confirm **megaloblastic anemia**).

Do the test results suggest a probable diagnosis? **NO**

YES

The doctor makes a list of possible diagnoses (the differential diagnosis).

TREATMENT IS STARTED

YES

Initial tests sometimes confirm a diagnosis (for example, **gallstones** from an ultrasound scan or **gout** from blood and joint fluid tests).

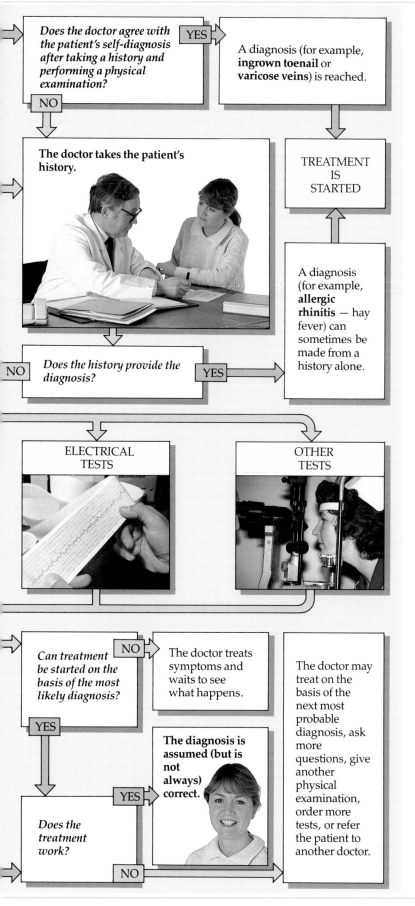

Does the doctor agree with the patient's self-diagnosis after taking a history and performing a physical examination?

YES → A diagnosis (for example, **ingrown toenail** or **varicose veins**) is reached.

NO

The doctor takes the patient's history.

TREATMENT IS STARTED

Does the history provide the diagnosis?

NO   **YES** → A diagnosis (for example, **allergic rhinitis** — hay fever) can sometimes be made from a history alone.

ELECTRICAL TESTS

OTHER TESTS

Can treatment be started on the basis of the most likely diagnosis?   **NO** → The doctor treats symptoms and waits to see what happens.

The doctor may treat on the basis of the next most probable diagnosis, ask more questions, give another physical examination, order more tests, or refer the patient to another doctor.

YES

The diagnosis is assumed (but is not always) correct.

Does the treatment work?   **YES** →

NO

changed dramatically from the days when X-rays were the mainstay; they now provide many different means of obtaining two- or three-dimensional pictures of the internal organs. In addition, the images generated can be made more detailed and informative by computer analysis and enhancement.

Today, many tests are noninvasive, which means that the patient is not subjected to any discomfort from the insertion of a needle, tube, or other device into the body. Some of the newer imaging procedures use sound waves, magnetic waves, or radio waves to provide pictures of internal body structures.

Are laboratory results reliable?

Because laboratories are equipped with expensive and elaborate hardware, the assumption is that they provide information that is invariably correct. In practice, this is not always the case. The interpretation of the results of laboratory tests requires both skill and experience.

Test results may be misleading for a number of reasons. First, the result may be wrong simply because a machine gives a false reading on the amount of a certain substance in the blood. Good laboratories run constant quality control tests, but unreliable apparatus or inexperienced technicians can give widely different results on repeated tests of a single specimen. Second, a test result that indicates a patient is outside the normal range for the measured variable does not necessarily mean that there is anything wrong with the patient (see UNDERSTANDING TEST RESULTS on page 15).

So, while many medical tests are highly accurate, in general they should be regarded as no more than a means of helping to confirm, or reject, your doctor's working diagnosis.

Doubtful diagnoses

What, then, does the doctor do when the results of your tests are returned and seem to indicate a particular disorder?

If the test results confirm the doctor's working diagnosis, nothing more needs to be done; the picture is consistent and the diagnosis is clear.

If, however, there is any doubt or uncertainty, or the diagnosis is grave (cancer or HIV infection, for example), the next step is to repeat the test to exclude the possibility of laboratory error. If necessary, the doctor may ask that the test be performed using a different technique to confirm the abnormality.

In addition, when the diagnosis is based more on the doctor's opinion than on clear test results, the patient may reasonably ask for a second opinion from another doctor. This is especially important when the possibility of an elective operation – that is, one done as a non-emergency procedure – is under discussion. Some doctors tend to be more interventionist than others; they believe in the old maxim "when in doubt take it out." Others are by temperament more cautious. Given that few operations have a 100 percent success rate and most involve some risk, it is preferable that the diagnosis be firmly established before surgery is decided upon.

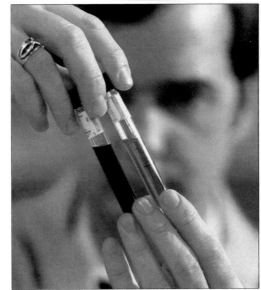

Laboratory tests
A wide range of diagnostic tests are now available to the doctor. However, medical tests are only one part of the process of diagnosis. They should not be regarded as more than a means of helping to confirm, or disprove, your doctor's ideas based on his or her other observations.

THE VALUE OF AN EARLY DIAGNOSIS

As recently as 20 years ago, many doctors had reservations about the value of performing regular physical examinations on people who felt healthy and had no symptoms. Attitudes have changed, however, as studies show that, among certain high-risk groups, screening tests detect disease earlier.

Computers and diagnosis
Doctors are using computers more than ever as diagnostic tools. It is possible to enter information about a patient's symptoms, signs, and laboratory results into a specially programmed computer. The computer then uses data banks of information from thousands of patients to calculate the probabilities of the different possible diagnoses using a process of "pattern recognition" similar to the doctor's. Here, the doctor is asking the patient a series of questions to help diagnose the cause of back pain.

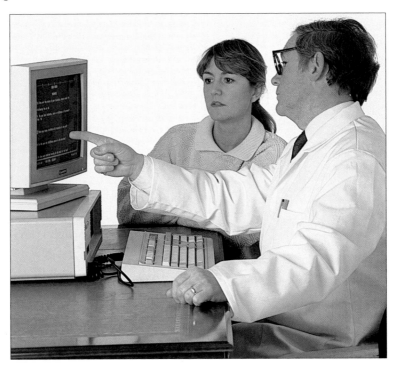

UNDERSTANDING TEST RESULTS

Many medical tests measure features of the body that vary widely even among healthy people. The manner in which these variables differ from person to person nearly always conforms to a fairly standard distribution. For example, if 100 men were stopped on the street and their heights were measured, the results would look something like the "people graph" illustrated at right. Other measurements – such as those for blood pressure or blood cholesterol – would provide similarly shaped graphs.

The reason doctors are interested in these features is that people who fall at the very ends of the range are more likely to have something wrong with them than those in the middle. For example, excessive or diminutive height may be caused by a pituitary gland disorder. Thus, people whose test results fall outside the normal range may undergo more tests.

It should be realized that a test measurement that is outside the normal range does not necessarily mean there is anything wrong with you. You may score a "high" or "low" result simply as a result of biological variability.

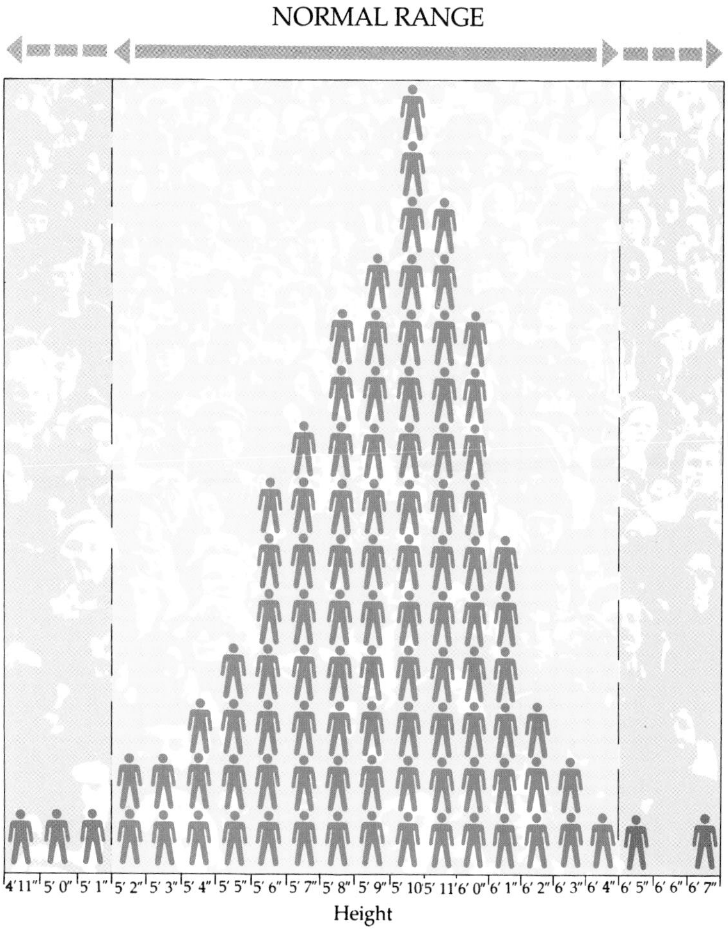

NORMAL RANGE

Height

An ideal screening test for a disease:

♦ Is both specific and sensitive. This means that, when the result indicates a disease, the disease is consistently present; there are few or no "false positive" test results. And, when the test result excludes the disease, the disease is consistently absent; there are few or no "false negative" test results.

♦ Has a reasonably high detection rate. For example, there is little reason to screen Americans for leprosy because so few have been exposed to the disease.

♦ Can be followed with an effective treatment for that disease. Detecting high blood pressure has been shown to be effective, because treatment is simple and prevents the occurrence of stroke or other complications, such as heart failure. By contrast, the detection of lung cancer through the use of chest X-rays is of less value because even in the early stages the disease is curable by surgery or radiation therapy only in rare cases.

Each year the number of screening tests has increased. This is especially true in the early detection of cancers.

How reliable are "do-it-yourself" diagnoses?

Few medical diagnoses can be made with 100 percent certainty immediately, and laboratory and other diagnostic tests require interpretation. All medical diagnoses require a combination of factual information and a careful assessment based on experience. That is why it is in the patient's best interests to leave the complex question of a final diagnosis to his or her doctor.

INVESTIGATING THE BODY SYSTEMS

Our bodies can be regarded as a collection of interdependent, but to some extent self-contained, systems, each with its own role or roles in the overall functioning of the body. The cardiovascular system, for example, circulates blood through the body, and the digestive system extracts and processes nutrients from food. The reproductive system produces ova (eggs), sperm, and the sex hormones that are responsible for reproduction. Many symptoms strongly suggest a disorder of a certain body system: this is why, after taking a medical history, doctors often concentrate on investigating one or two specific functions of a particular system. In this section, the main body systems are reviewed one by one, with cross-references to the procedures that are performed for diagnosing diseases of each system.

THE DIGESTIVE SYSTEM

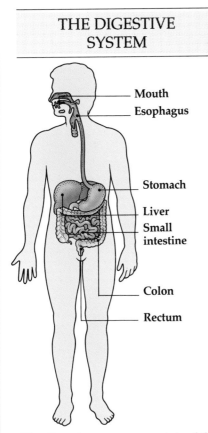

Mouth
Esophagus

Stomach

Liver
Small intestine

Colon

Rectum

The digestive system consists of the alimentary tract – a continuous tube from the mouth to the anus that includes the esophagus, stomach, small intestine, colon, and rectum – along with three associated organs, the liver, gallbladder, and pancreas. Nutrients from food entering the tract are absorbed from the intestines into the lymphatic system and bloodstream and processed by the liver. Secretions from the stomach and pancreas, and bile from the liver (which is stored temporarily in the gallbladder), assist in the breakdown of food. Solid waste products are conveyed via the colon to the rectum and expelled via the anus.

Symptoms of digestive tract disorders may include dry mouth, excessive salivation, difficulty swallowing, heartburn, excess gas, abdominal pain or swelling, general malaise, vomiting, diarrhea, constipation, weight loss, or pain or bleeding during defecation.

Investigating digestive disorders

After taking a history of the problem, your doctor performs a physical examination (see THE DIGESTIVE SYSTEM, page 29), which may include inspection of the mouth, palpation and percussion of the abdomen, and a rectal examination. PLAIN X-RAY EXAMINATIONS (page 39) can give information about abnormalities in the digestive tract that can be supplemented by BARIUM X-RAY EXAMINATIONS (page 44), including barium meal and barium enema.

Endoscopic techniques are particularly useful for investigating digestive system problems such as ulcerative conditions and gastrointestinal polyps. They include ESOPHAGOSCOPY AND GASTRODUODENOSCOPY (page 70) for examining the upper portion of the tract, and COLONOSCOPY (page 71) and SIGMOIDOSCOPY AND PROCTOSCOPY (page 72) for problems lower down. ERCP (page 47) is used to examine the ducts from the liver, gallbladder, and pancreas.

Other relevant imaging techniques include ULTRASOUND SCANNING (page 60), which is especially useful for looking at the gallbladder, liver, and pancreas; CT SCANNING (page 48); and MAGNETIC RESONANCE IMAGING (page 54). RADIONUCLIDE SCANNING (page 50) can be used to view the liver and pancreas.

Tissue samples can be taken via an endoscope or via a needle or capsule (see BIOPSIES, page 100, and JEJUNAL BIOPSY, page 135) and examined under a microscope. Fecal samples can be chemically tested for blood or fats (see FECAL TESTS, page 111), cultured for organisms, or examined under the microscope (see CULTURE AND MICROSCOPY, page 114).

Other tests relevant to digestive system disorders include LIVER AND KIDNEY FUNCTION TESTS (page 110), measurement of BLOOD ENZYMES (page 109), the GASTRIC ACID SECRETION TEST (page 133), and the XYLOSE TOLERANCE TEST (page 141).

THE RESPIRATORY SYSTEM

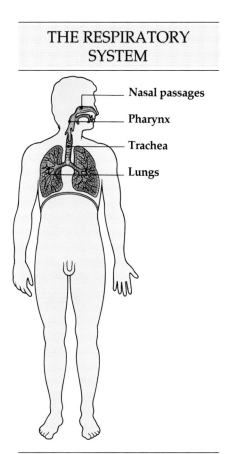

Nasal passages

Pharynx

Trachea

Lungs

THE CARDIOVASCULAR SYSTEM

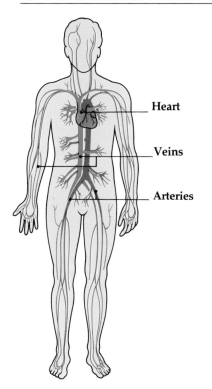

Heart

Veins

Arteries

The respiratory system consists of the passages through which air is conveyed to the lungs and the air passages and sacs in the lungs themselves. Oxygen in the air is breathed into the lungs and is absorbed into the blood; waste carbon dioxide is transferred from the blood to the lungs and is breathed out.

Symptoms of respiratory system disorders include sneezing, stuffiness, sore throat, coughing, shortness of breath, wheezing, chest pain, coughing up blood, a raised temperature, and difficulty breathing at rest or during exertion.

Investigating respiratory disorders

After taking the medical history, the doctor performs a physical examination (see THE RESPIRATORY SYSTEM, page 30). The examination includes listening to the lungs, and percussion and palpation of the chest. The flow of air into and out of the lungs and the lung volume may also be measured (see SPIROMETRY, page 139). Swabs from the throat or a sample of sputum (phlegm) may also be taken (see CULTURE AND MICROSCOPY, page 114).

The throat can be examined by tongue depressor, nasopharyngoscopy, or LARYNGOSCOPY (page 74), and the airways in the lungs by BRONCHOSCOPY (page 75). Samples of bronchial and lung tissue can be taken for microscopic examination.

Imaging techniques used to examine the lungs include PLAIN X-RAY EXAMINATIONS (page 39), BRONCHOGRAPHY (page 129), CT SCANNING (page 48), and MAGNETIC RESONANCE IMAGING (page 54). The blood supply to the lungs can be imaged by pulmonary ANGIOGRAPHY (page 45) and the distribution of blood by RADIONUCLIDE SCANNING (page 50). Samples of blood may be taken to measure the levels of oxygen and carbon dioxide (see BLOOD GASES, page 108).

The cardiovascular system consists of the heart and the blood vessels. The heart is a powerful muscle that pumps blood, via the blood vessels called arteries, to all parts of the body. Blood is transported back to the heart by veins.

Symptoms of cardiovascular disease include chest pain, breathlessness, palpitations, swelling of the ankles and other areas, tiredness, dizziness, fainting, pain in the legs when walking, and, occasionally, pain that is felt in the jaw, throat, arm, or wrist.

Investigating cardiovascular disorders

When the doctor takes a medical history, he or she concentrates on such points as exercise tolerance. The doctor will also ask about hypertension (high blood pressure), smoking, diabetes, cholesterol level, rheumatic fever, alcohol intake, and your family history. During the physical examination (see HEART AND CIRCULATION, page 30), measurement of the pulse and blood pressure are particularly important, and the doctor will listen carefully to your heart through a stethoscope.

ELECTROCARDIOGRAPHY (page 82) is one of the most common tests for investigating the heart. Imaging techniques to look for structural or functional abnormalities of the heart include PLAIN X-RAY EXAMINATIONS (page 39), ECHOCARDIOGRAPHY (page 64), RADIONUCLIDE SCANNING (page 50), PET SCANNING (page 52), and SPECT examination (page 51). ANGIOGRAPHY (page 45) and DOPPLER SCANNING (page 65) can be used to view blood flow through both the heart and arteries. CARDIAC CATHETERIZATION (page 130) allows the doctor to take pressure readings from within the chambers of the heart. Measurement of BLOOD ENZYMES (page 109) can also be relevant to heart disease. Another technique used to diagnose blood vessel disease is VENOGRAPHY (page 141).

THE NERVOUS SYSTEM

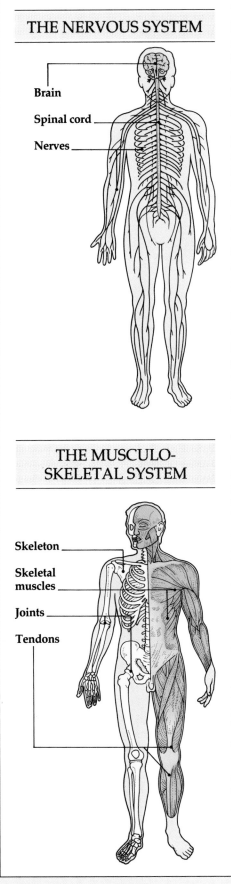

Brain

Spinal cord

Nerves

The nervous system consists of the brain and spinal cord, and the nerves that fan out from them to the body. The brain and spinal cord make up the central nervous system; the remaining nerves constitute the peripheral nervous system.

The nervous system is the body's principal control, communications, and information storage system. Information is continuously carried from sense organs via sensory nerves to the spinal cord and brain, where the information is analyzed. Responses are initiated by messages sent along motor nerves to the muscles and along autonomic nerves to glands and other organs.

Symptoms of nervous system disorder include sensory disturbances or loss of sensation, muscle weakness, paralysis or clumsiness, difficulties with memory, speech, or walking, disturbances of consciousness, tremor, seizures, headaches, or pain anywhere in the body.

Investigating nervous system disorders

The history of the illness, and the physical examination (see THE NERVOUS SYSTEM, page 32), including an assessment of speech, movement, sensory ability, and reflexes, can give clues to the nature of a problem.

Examination of the inside of the eyes by OPHTHALMOSCOPY (page 80) and by a VISUAL FIELD TEST (page 141) can indicate any problems with the retina, optic nerve, or brain itself.

Diagnostic tests used to look at the brain include CT SCANNING (page 48), MAGNETIC RESONANCE IMAGING (page 54), cerebral ANGIOGRAPHY (page 45), PET SCANNING (page 52), and ELECTROENCEPHALOGRAPHY (page 86). NERVE CONDUCTION STUDIES (page 136) and evoked responses (page 87) may be used to test nerve pathways.

If an infection of the fluid that bathes the brain and spinal cord is suspected, LUMBAR PUNCTURE (page 99) may be performed.

THE MUSCULO-SKELETAL SYSTEM

Skeleton

Skeletal muscles

Joints

Tendons

The musculoskeletal system consists of the skeleton, the skeletal muscles and their tendons, the joints, and the ligaments, which serve to bind joints together.

The skeleton provides the body with a framework and means of support. The joints between the bones allow movement, initiated by contractions of the skeletal muscles.

Symptoms and signs of musculoskeletal disorders include muscle pain or weakness, pain and stiffness during movement, back pain, bone deformity, and joint swelling.

Investigating musculoskeletal disorders

The investigation of musculoskeletal disorders begins with taking a history and performing a physical examination (see the LOCOMOTOR SYSTEM, page 33), which includes an assessment of joint movement and muscle strength and an inspection for any bone or joint swelling, tenderness, and/or deformity.

PLAIN X-RAY EXAMINATIONS (page 39), which can reveal fractures or joint abnormalities, are among the most useful tests for skeletal disorders. RADIONUCLIDE SCANNING (page 50) may be helpful in diagnosing some types of bone disease. The inside of the joints can be inspected by arthroscopy (page 77) and fluid from the joints can be obtained by JOINT ASPIRATION (page 99).

BIOPSIES (page 100) of bone and muscle may be taken. Blood tests relevant to musculoskeletal disorders include measurement of creatine phosphokinase (see BLOOD ENZYMES, page 109), URIC ACID MEASUREMENT (page 140) in the diagnosis of gout, CALCIUM MEASUREMENT (page 129) in the diagnosis of bone disease, RHEUMATOID FACTOR MEASUREMENT (page 138) in the diagnosis of rheumatoid arthritis, and an ANTINUCLEAR ANTIBODIES TEST (page 129) in the diagnosis of systemic lupus erythematosus or other connective tissue diseases.

THE KIDNEYS AND URINARY SYSTEM

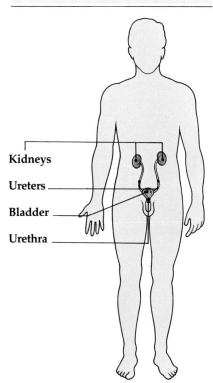

Kidneys

Ureters

Bladder

Urethra

The kidneys maintain the internal chemical balance of the body by removing unnecessary substances (such as urea, creatinine, and metabolized drugs) and variable amounts of water and salts from the blood and excreting them in the urine. Urine passes via the ureters to the bladder, where it is stored until it is expelled from the body.

Symptoms of kidney and urinary tract disorders may include pain in the groin, pelvic region, or lower back, pain during urination, difficulty urinating, cloudy or blood-stained urine, incontinence, urinary frequency, and fever.

Investigating urinary system disorders

After taking a medical history, the doctor may perform a physical examination (see THE URINARY SYSTEM, page 34). CHEMICAL TESTS (page 108) on the blood and urine, including kidney function tests such as UREA NITROGEN MEASUREMENT (page 140)

and the CREATININE CLEARANCE TEST (page 131), can assist in the diagnosis of kidney disease. The urine may also be inspected for color and cloudiness, tested for the presence of blood, protein, and sugar, cultured for infectious organisms, and inspected under a microscope for crystals, bacteria, red blood cells, and white blood cells (see CULTURE AND MICROSCOPY, page 114).

The entire urinary tract can be imaged by ULTRASOUND SCANNING (page 60) or PYELOGRAPHY (page 47); the blood supply to the kidneys can be imaged by renal ANGIOGRAPHY (page 45). More information about the kidneys can be obtained by CT SCANNING (page 48), RADIONUCLIDE SCANNING (page 50), and BIOPSIES (page 100). Other relevant investigations may include KIDNEY STONE ANALYSIS (page 135). The inside of the bladder can be viewed by CYSTOURETHROSCOPY (page 76) and bladder function can be assessed by CYSTOMETRY (page 131).

THE ENDOCRINE SYSTEM

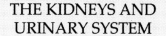

Pituitary gland

Thyroid gland

Parathyroid glands

Adrenal glands

Pancreas

Ovaries (female)

Testes (male)

The primary endocrine glands are the adrenal, thyroid, and parathyroid glands, and the pancreas, testes, and ovaries. All the glands secrete hormones; these chemical messengers help control body processes, such as metabolism and sexual maturation. The master gland is the pituitary gland, located in the brain, which secretes hormones that regulate most of the other glands.

Because the endocrine system affects all aspects of body function, disorders may include such diverse signs and symptoms as fatigue, thirst, excess urine production, slow or premature sexual maturation, excess body hair, weight gain or loss, changes in body fat distribution, anxiety, and skin changes.

Investigating endocrine disorders

If a doctor suspects an endocrine disorder, special tests may be performed to confirm the diagnosis.

Most hormones can be measured in the blood, and abnormal levels of pituitary or other hormones can provide conclusive evidence of an endocrine disorder (see ADRENOCORTICOTROPIC HORMONE MEASUREMENT, page 128; ALDOSTERONE MEASUREMENT, page 128; ANTIDIURETIC HORMONE MEASUREMENT, page 128; CALCITONIN MEASUREMENT, page 129; CORTISOL MEASUREMENT, page 131; ESTROGEN MEASUREMENT, page 132; FOLLICLE-STIMULATING HORMONE MEASUREMENT, page 132; GLUCAGON MEASUREMENT, page 133; GROWTH HORMONE MEASUREMENT, page 133; INSULIN MEASUREMENT, page 134; LUTEINIZING HORMONE MEASUREMENT, page 135; PARATHYROID HORMONE MEASUREMENT, page 136; PROLACTIN MEASUREMENT, page 137; and THYROID HORMONES MEASUREMENT, page 140). The diagnosis of diabetes mellitus (caused by a pancreatic disorder) is confirmed by measuring the level of glucose in the blood.

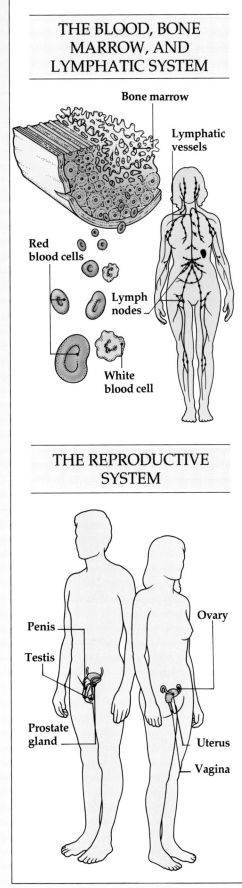

THE BLOOD, BONE MARROW, AND LYMPHATIC SYSTEM

Bone marrow

Lymphatic vessels

Red blood cells

Lymph nodes

White blood cell

THE REPRODUCTIVE SYSTEM

Penis

Testis

Prostate gland

Ovary

Uterus

Vagina

Most of the cells in blood – the red and white blood cells and the cells called platelets – are formed in the marrow of flat bones. Some white cells are made in the lymph glands. The red cells carry oxygen in blood, and the white cells help defend the body against infection. The platelets form a clot when a blood vessel is injured and bleeding occurs. Many other important blood components are made in the liver.

Many types of white cells move between the blood and the lymphatic system, an interconnected network of lymph nodes. The lymphatic system is the main defense against infection; its white cells form antibodies that kill invading microbes, while its nodes also act as filters, isolating invading microbes and matter made up of minute particles such as soot and dusts.

Symptoms of blood and bone marrow disorders may include weakness, tiredness, and breath-lessness, an increased tendency to infections, and bleeding tendencies. Symptoms and signs of lymphatic system disease include swelling of the lymph nodes in the neck and groin, or fever.

Investigating blood and lymphatic disorders

Blood and bone marrow disorders are investigated by WHOLE BLOOD TESTS (see page 102), including counts of the cells in blood, a BLOOD SMEAR (page 103), and sometimes a BONE MARROW BIOPSY (page 129). More tests may be needed to clarify the causes of particular blood disorders such as pernicious anemia. BLOOD CLOTTING TESTS (page 104) may be performed to investigate bleeding disorders. BONE MARROW BIOPSY (page 129), LYMPH NODE BIOPSY (page 136), and MAGNETIC RESONANCE IMAGING (page 54) or CT SCANNING (page 48) are used to investigate lymphatic system disease.

The male and female reproductive systems have complementary roles. Symptoms of reproductive system disorders in the male may include painful urination or penile discharge, lumps or ulcers on the penis, swellings in the scrotum, or a painful or nodular testicle. In women, disorders may include vaginal discharge or irritation, ulceration on the external genitals, abdominal or pelvic pain, absent or abnormally heavy periods, or pain during intercourse.

Investigating reproductive system disorders

After taking a medical history, the doctor examines the reproductive organs by inspection and palpation. In women, the doctor performs a pelvic examination (page 29).

Vaginal or penile discharges (or scrapings and smears from the external genitals) may be analyzed by CULTURE AND MICROSCOPY (page 114). The doctor may order specific tests for some sexually transmitted diseases (see SYPHILIS, TESTS FOR, page 139 and GONORRHEA, TESTS FOR, page 133).

The female reproductive organs can be inspected further by COLPOSCOPY (page 77), LAPAROSCOPY (page 74), ULTRASOUND SCANNING (page 60), and HYSTEROSALPINGOGRAPHY (page 134). A CERVICAL (PAP) SMEAR (page 97) may be done and a sample of the cervix taken by CERVICAL PUNCH BIOPSY (page 130). A sample of the uterine lining may be taken by ENDOMETRIAL BIOPSY (page 101).

Other investigations that may be relevant to reproductive system disorders include PROSTATE GLAND BIOPSY (page 100), ESTROGEN MEASUREMENT (page 132), PROGESTERONE MEASUREMENT (page 137), TESTOSTERONE MEASUREMENT (page 140), IMPOTENCE TESTS (page 134), LUTEINIZING HORMONE MEASUREMENT (page 135), FOLLICLE-STIMULATING HORMONE MEASUREMENT (page 132), and SEMEN ANALYSIS (page 139).

THE SKIN

The skin is the body's protective covering. It consists of a thin, waterproof, outer layer, the epidermis, and a thicker underlying layer, the dermis, which contains blood vessels, connective and elastic tissue, sweat glands, and many sensory receptors. Symptoms of skin disorders include pimples, rashes, lumps, spots, blistering, itching, dryness, scaling, or ulceration.

THE EYE AND VISUAL SYSTEM

The visual system has two parts – optical and neurological. The optical portion consists of the cornea at the front of the eye and the internal lens, which focus light from the objects you observe to the retina lining the back of the eyeball. The retina represents the beginning of the neurological portion of the visual system. It produces electrochemical signals that pass along the optic nerve to the nerves that lead to the back of the brain, where the signals are transmitted and interpreted to produce an image. Symptoms of eye and visual problems include eye pain or irritation, watering, dryness, blurred vision, or partial or total vision loss.

THE EAR AND HEARING SYSTEM

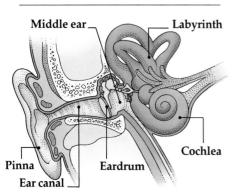

Middle ear — Labyrinth

Cochlea

Pinna — Eardrum

Ear canal

Investigating skin disorders

Most skin disorders can be diagnosed from their appearance. Diagnosis may be assisted or confirmed by BIOPSIES (page 100) followed by MICROSCOPY (page 114) to look for fungi or for changes in skin structure or changes in individual cells, by SKIN REACTION TESTS (page 139), by CULTURE (page 114) for bacteria, and by WOOD'S LIGHT EXAMINATION (page 141) for fungal infection. Skin samples can also be subjected to IMMUNOLOGICAL TESTS (page 112).

Investigating eye and visual disorders

After taking a history, the outer portion of the eyes and eyelids are inspected (see THE EYE, page 34). For visual problems, VISUAL ACUITY AND REFRACTION TESTS (page 141) may be used to determine the power of

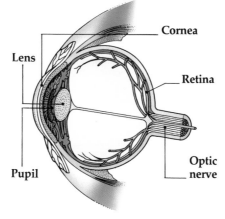

Lens

Cornea

Retina

Pupil

Optic nerve

The ear consists of the pinna, external ear canal, eardrum, middle-ear cavity, and the inner ear, which contains the cochlea and the labyrinth. Sound vibrations are conveyed to the cochlea via the eardrum and three tiny bones in the middle ear. There they are converted into electrical signals, which are sent via the acoustic nerve to the brain for interpretation. Symptoms of ear and hearing disorders include earache, ear fullness, discharge, ringing in the ears, and nausea, vomiting, and vertigo.

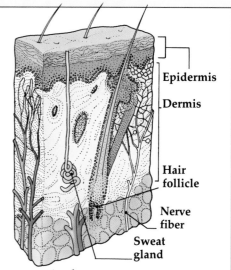

Epidermis

Dermis

Hair follicle

Nerve fiber

Sweat gland

corrective lenses. COLOR VISION TESTS (page 131) may also be performed.

Special EYE EXAMINATIONS (page 78) include a SLIT-LAMP EXAMINATION (page 78) to examine the external eye, assessments of ocular movement and alignment, a PUPILLARY REFLEX TEST (page 137), APPLANATION TONOMETRY (page 79) to test for glaucoma, OPHTHALMOSCOPY (page 80) to examine the retina, and FLUORESCEIN ANGIOGRAPHY (page 81) to examine the retinal vessels.

More specific tests on the eye include a FLUORESCEIN EYE STAIN (page 132), OCULAR ULTRASOUND (page 80), a VISUAL FIELD TEST (page 141), and SCHIRMER'S TEST (page 138). MAGNETIC RESONANCE IMAGING (page 54) or CT SCANNING (page 48) may be performed to look for suspected orbital or brain disease affecting vision.

Investigating ear and hearing disorders

After taking a history, the doctor examines the outer ear, ear canal, and eardrum with an otoscope (see THE EAR, page 34). A variety of HEARING TESTS (page 88) may be performed, including tuning fork tests (page 89), AUDIOMETRY (page 90), IMPEDANCE AUDIOMETRY (page 90), and SPEECH AUDIOMETRY (page 90). Other tests relevant to hearing and balance problems include the CALORIC TEST (page 129) and ELECTRONYSTAGMOGRAPHY (page 132).

CHAPTER TWO

THE DOCTOR'S EXAMINATION

INTRODUCTION

TAKING THE PATIENT'S HISTORY

THE PHYSICAL EXAMINATION

THE MEDICAL CONSULTATION consists of two parts. The first is the taking of the patient's medical history, which gives the doctor some idea of what the problem is likely to be. The second is the physical examination, which confirms or corrects the doctor's initial impressions. The doctor often spends at least as much, or more, time taking the medical history as conducting the physical examination. Both parts of the consultation are described in this chapter to give you a thorough understanding of what thought processes the doctor goes through to reach a diagnosis.

The first section, TAKING THE PATIENT'S HISTORY, gives examples of the questions your doctor may ask during history-taking, and how your answers can provide vital clues to the diagnosis. There are many instances in which a brief description of the problem, as told in your own words, is sufficient information for the doctor to reach a fairly firm diagnosis. However, in other cases, it is necessary for the doctor to ask more specific questions about the precise nature and duration of an illness, and the order in which the symptoms appeared. You may be asked questions about your life-style, occupation, any past illnesses and treatments, and about your family's medical history,

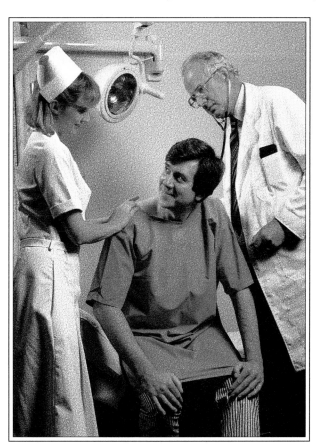

especially that of parents and siblings. A family history of a particular disease may increase the probability of such a condition developing in you. Keeping a record of these details may also alert a doctor to a patient's need for screening tests. If, for example, several of your relatives had bowel cancer, your doctor may recommend that you have periodic tests to make sure that you do not have a symptomless tumor.

Before beginning THE PHYSICAL EXAMINATION, your doctor already has (from the medical history) a fairly good idea of which system of the body is affected. This section explains the methods doctors commonly use to examine the digestive system, heart and circulation, respiratory system, nervous system, locomotor system, eyes and ears, and urinary system. However, because an illness can affect more than one part of the body, your doctor will probably examine all of your body systems. The problems that can be the most difficult to diagnose are those with nonspecific symptoms, such as feelings of being tired or "under the weather." The problem usually requires a more lengthy investigation if the doctor has not reached a working diagnosis by the time he or she has taken a medical history and completed a full physical examination.

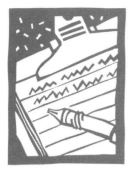

TAKING THE PATIENT'S HISTORY

I N AN ERA OF increasingly high-tech medicine, it is sometimes hard to believe that taking a patient's medical history is still the most significant part of the diagnostic process. Your medical history remains the most important diagnostic indicator of disease because it points the way (among the myriad tests available) to the procedures that will prove to be most informative and beneficial.

The consultation
History-taking is an important diagnostic tool. Don't hold back information and don't attempt to make your own diagnosis. Do try to give a clear description of your problem.

A patient's medical history is a record of everything that is relevant to his or her health. The medical history includes details of the current problem, any previous illnesses, and the patient's social, occupational, and family background. When talking to your doctor about your medical history, don't withhold anything and don't hesitate to explain your symptoms in the words that best describe the way you feel.

The answer to a single question opens up a wide range of diagnostic possibilities. Because there are so many different

possibilities, your doctor will take into account the influence of probabilities, knowing which conditions are most common and therefore most likely. A series of well-worded questions (and the subsequent answers from the patient) will indicate the most promising avenue to the doctor, who will follow this route for as long as the responses are consistent with his or her initial impression.

FAMILY HISTORY

History-taking – the ongoing dialogue between you and your doctor – is important to the diagnostic process. What may begin as a casual conversation can evolve gradually into a more detailed question-and-answer period about your own and your family's health habits. Effective history-taking is based on medical knowledge and is impossible without it. Doctors who can take a thorough, revealing history have mastered a fine art.

Information about your relatives' illnesses or cause of death is also important to your doctor's diagnosis. Many diseases run in families, even when there is no obvious genetic reason. A family history of certain conditions, such as coronary heart disease, diabetes mellitus, high blood pressure, gout, or ulcers, may increase the probability of the condition developing in you. Your doctor may want to perform tests to rule out this possibility at an early stage.

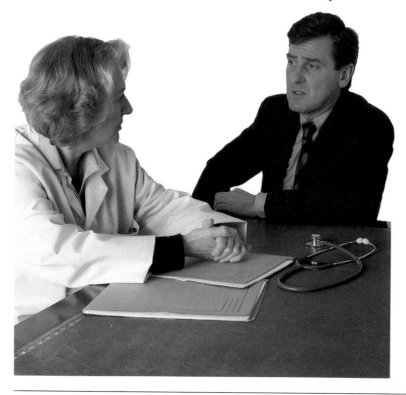

WHY YOUR FAMILY HISTORY IS IMPORTANT

The medical history of even distant relatives can have a bearing on the diagnostic process. For example, Sean, a 6-year-old boy, had painful, swollen joints. During a conversation with Sean's parents, the doctor learned that a cousin and probably a great uncle suffered from the genetic bleeding disorder hemophilia (see family tree below). This information pointed almost immediately to Sean's diagnosis – he, too, had hemophilia and was suffering from bleeding into his joints, which was causing the pain and swelling.

Sean's mother and some other female relatives are probable carriers of the hemophilia gene. They do not suffer from the disease themselves. They do, though, pass on the gene to some of their sons, in whom hemophilia develops, and to some of their daughters, who become carriers.

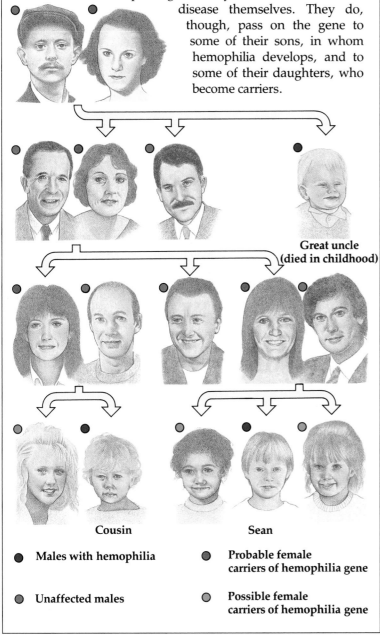

**Great uncle
(died in childhood)**

Cousin   **Sean**

● **Males with hemophilia**   ● **Probable female
carriers of hemophilia gene**

● **Unaffected males**   ● **Possible female
carriers of hemophilia gene**

PREVIOUS ILLNESSES

Your doctor will ask you about any previous illnesses, injuries, and hospital admissions, from childhood onward, and will try to get an idea of the general quality of your past health.

The doctor will then consider your current complaint. At this point, he or she will probably have an idea of what the problem is, and will continue the conversation with specific questions based on his or her experience and knowledge of the likely disorder.

LIFE-STYLE

Life-style can have a tremendous impact on your health. Your doctor may ask you questions about any of the following aspects of your life to further develop his or her understanding of your habits.

Alcohol and diet

Excessive use of alcohol can cause liver damage; inflammation of the stomach, pancreas, or heart muscle; vitamin and nutritional deficiency; certain forms of anemia; and brain damage. Don't be embarrassed or afraid to tell your doctor how much you drink.

Many people overeat and choose unhealthy foods, leading to high cholesterol levels in the blood and an increased risk of the serious arterial disease atherosclerosis. Tell your doctor if you follow a radical or restricted diet, and be honest about your regular eating habits.

Drugs

There are serious risks involved in the intravenous taking of drugs and the sharing of needles. The risks include bloodstream infections with fungal and bacterial organisms, and infection with potentially lethal viruses such as the hepatitis B virus or HIV (the AIDS virus). It is also important to tell your doctor if you use prescription drugs or any substances such as cocaine or marijuana.

WHAT YOUR DOCTOR SHOULD KNOW ABOUT YOU

During your consultation, be sure to tell your doctor anything that might be relevant to your current condition. This includes any previous illness your doctor may not know about, all symptoms (even those that seem unconnected to your current problem), allergies, medications you take, alcohol intake, and recent travel abroad.

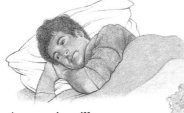

Any previous illnesses
Past disorders may shed light on your present condition.

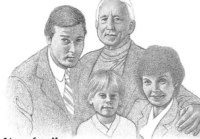

Your current symptoms
Give as clear a description as possible of your symptoms.

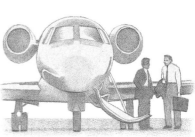

Travel abroad
If you have been abroad recently, you may have picked up an infection, such as malaria or hepatitis.

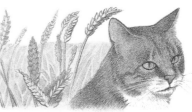

Allergies
Don't forget to tell your doctor about any allergies to pollens, house-dust mites, drugs, antibiotics, or foods.

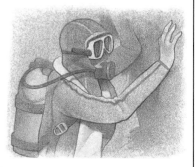

Your family
The state of health or cause of death of close relatives can be significant.

Medications
You could be experiencing side effects from drugs. Tell your doctor about any medication you have been taking.

Sports
Certain sports, such as scuba diving and mountain climbing, can affect your health and may be relevant.

Exercise, sleep, and smoking

The amount and type of exercise you do is very important. Obesity and poor tolerance to exercise can give your doctor vital clues to such conditions as coronary heart disease or obstructive disease of the airways in the lungs.

Disturbances of the normal sleep pattern are common in depression, anxiety, and conditions causing persistent pain.

Many conditions are known to be related to smoking, including bronchitis and emphysema; cancers of the larynx, lung, esophagus, mouth and pancreas; coronary heart disease; peptic ulcer; arterial disease; and stroke. Ask your doctor to help you quit smoking now.

Sex

Your doctor may ask if you are heterosexual, homosexual, or bisexual and if you are monogamous or have multiple partners. Your sexual orientation influences your doctor's consideration of symptoms that may occur as a result of sexually transmitted disease.

OCCUPATION

Many jobs involve hazards to health. Some of these hazards are obvious; others may not affect your health until years later. Not only is your current job relevant – work that you performed many years ago can sometimes be responsible for a current disease. A history of employment in an asbestos-processing plant, for example, is likely to be highly relevant to a current problem with persistent cough and breathlessness.

Job satisfaction

Your doctor may also ask you about your satisfaction with your work. Does your job interest you or do you work only for the money? Do you get along with your colleagues? Are there stress factors, both physical and psychological, that may be affecting your health?

Occupational disease
Diseases and disorders related to occupation are estimated to affect more than 100,000 Americans annually. For example, a welder (below) may be at increased risk of eye injuries. Always tell your doctor about your present and any past occupations.

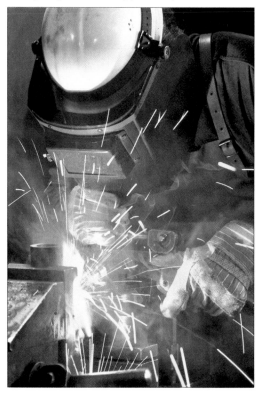

IS YOUR JOB AFFECTING YOUR HEALTH?

Some occupations carry an obvious risk of physical injury. Others have less apparent dangers. Exposure to the following as a result of your work may be a cause of illness, which is why your doctor may ask you questions about your occupation during the history-taking.

♦ **Industrial solvents** Industrial solvents can cause allergies or dermatitis. They can also damage your kidneys or liver.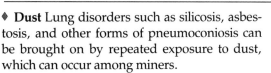

♦ **Dust** Lung disorders such as silicosis, asbestosis, and other forms of pneumoconiosis can be brought on by repeated exposure to dust, which can occur among miners.

♦ **Heat** Heat can cause muscle cramps, heat exhaustion, and heat stroke. Workers in metal-forming industries may be at risk.

♦ **Vibration to the hands** Repeated vibrations can damage the blood supply to the fingertips, and cause sensitivity to cold, arterial malfunction, and gangrene of the fingertips.

♦ **Pesticides** Pesticides may damage the kidneys, liver, nervous system, or sex glands (testicles or ovaries). Workers in agriculture or pesticide manufacture may be at risk.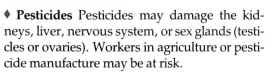

♦ **Noise** Impaired hearing can be the result of exposure to very loud noise, which can occur among people who work at airports.

♦ **Radiation** Cancer and damage to the skin, hair, and reproductive and blood-forming tissues are possible results of exposure. Workers in the nuclear industry may be exposed.

♦ **Contaminated water** Contact with, or drinking, infected water can cause leptospirosis, typhoid, and hepatitis. Workers in the water and sewage industries may be at risk.

♦ **Overcrowding and poor working conditions** Stress, smoking or drinking, illnesses such as peptic ulcer, and respiratory infections may be caused by poor working conditions.

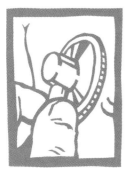

THE PHYSICAL EXAMINATION

BEFORE PERFORMING a physical examination, your doctor will have already made an assessment of your appearance and will probably have suspicions as to what is wrong. After you have been weighed and your blood pressure has been measured, the next step is a detailed physical examination based on those suspicions.

THE FACE AS AN INDICATOR OF DISEASE

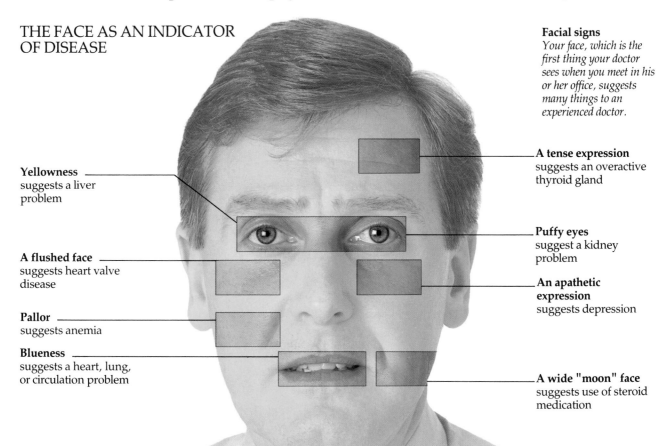

Facial signs
Your face, which is the first thing your doctor sees when you meet in his or her office, suggests many things to an experienced doctor.

Yellowness
suggests a liver problem

A flushed face
suggests heart valve disease

Pallor
suggests anemia

Blueness
suggests a heart, lung, or circulation problem

A tense expression
suggests an overactive thyroid gland

Puffy eyes
suggest a kidney problem

An apathetic expression
suggests depression

A wide "moon" face
suggests use of steroid medication

INSPECTION

Your doctor usually begins by asking you to undress and put on a paper gown or sheet. He or she may first examine your skin, checking for dryness, bruising, tiny red spots that suggest leakage from blood vessels, rashes, tumors, tattoos, and fluid under the skin.

If your doctor finds any of these features, new possibilities may be considered in conjunction with your medical history. The smallest detail may be important. For example, because tattooing is a means of transmitting blood-borne infection, a tattoo may indicate the source of a hepatitis B virus infection that has caused fever, jaundice, abdominal pain, and enlargement of the liver.

The doctor may also pinch your skin to check for loss of elasticity and to assess whether or not you have lost weight; look at your fingertips to see if they show the bulblike swelling, or clubbing, that is a feature of several serious conditions affecting the heart and lungs; take your temperature; and feel your groin and armpits for enlarged lymph nodes.

THE DIGESTIVE SYSTEM

To examine your digestive system, the doctor will first look into your mouth and note the appearance of your tongue and teeth and the smell of your breath.

The doctor will then ask you to lie down and will palpate your abdomen, feeling it carefully for tenderness, muscle resistance, any abnormal masses, and the lower edges of the liver and the spleen, which can be felt when they are enlarged. He or she also will want to know if you have any excess gas or liquid in the abdominal cavity and may tap your abdomen to check for any odd resonance or dull sounds.

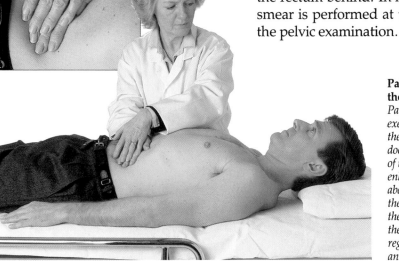

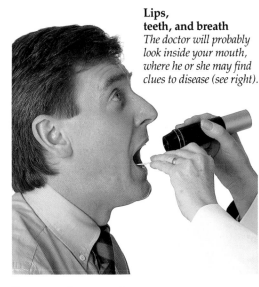

Lips, teeth, and breath
The doctor will probably look inside your mouth, where he or she may find clues to disease (see right).

Internal examination

The doctor will almost certainly perform a rectal examination using special disposable plastic gloves and a lubricating cream or jelly. Tumors of the prostate, rectum, and female reproductive organs are first suspected in this way. You will feel only a slight sensation much like when you move your bowels.

If you are a woman, a pelvic examination provides the doctor with important information about disorders of the urinary and genital organs. The doctor is concerned with visualizing the vagina and cervix and with feeling the uterus and ovaries in your pelvis through the walls of the vagina. The bladder can be felt at the front of the vagina, the wall of the rectum behind. In most cases, a Pap smear is performed at the same time as the pelvic examination.

Palpation of the abdomen
Palpation is done by exerting pressure with the flat of the hand. The doctor feels for any areas of tenderness, masses, or enlargement of the abdominal organs. Here, the doctor is examining the upper left quadrant of the abdomen, in the region of the stomach, for an enlarged spleen.

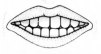
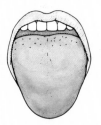

MEASURING BLOOD PRESSURE

Measuring blood pressure is a simple procedure that offers important insight into the state of your heart and blood vessels. The procedure measures the peak (systole) and trough (diastole) of the pressure wave produced in the arteries with each contraction of your heart muscle.

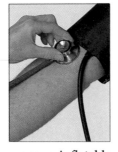

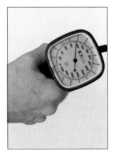

The doctor or nurse wraps an inflatable cuff firmly around the arm just above the elbow, connects it to a pressure gauge, and feels for your wrist pulse. The cuff is inflated until the pulse can no longer be felt at the wrist. It is then deflated slowly while the doctor listens for a pulse in the artery at the elbow. As the pressure in the cuff drops, sounds of the blood returning can be heard, first at the systolic pressure and then at the diastolic pressure. The measurement is read off the pressure gauge or mercury column. Electronic measuring devices are also available.

Blood pressure is measured in millimeters of mercury (mm Hg). A resting blood pressure higher than 150 mm Hg (systolic)/90 mm Hg (diastolic) is generally considered to be too high.

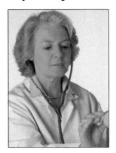

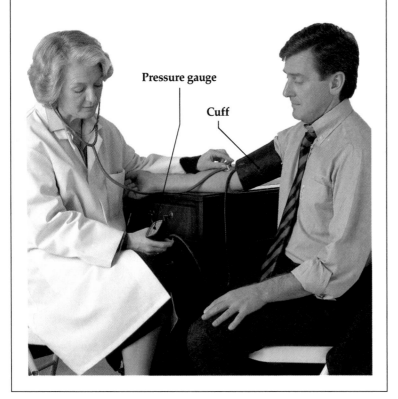

Pressure gauge

Cuff

HEART AND CIRCULATION

If the doctor suspects you have a heart or circulation problem, he or she will be especially interested in your pulse. The rate, rhythm, force, and regularity will be checked and your blood pressure will be taken at least twice during the consultation, perhaps once when you are lying down and once when sitting up.

The doctor will also want to note the position at which he or she can feel the lowest and outermost beat of your heart, which can indicate enlargement. The character of your heartbeat may be forceful and thrusting (indicating a possibly overloaded heart) or relatively weak and tapping (which suggests a poor flow into the main pumping chamber).

It is sometimes possible to feel "thrills" (fluttering sensations) over the heart; these are caused by an abnormal turbulence in blood flow. Your doctor will consider this abnormality in conjunction with any abnormal heart sounds (murmurs) he or she hears through the stethoscope, which may indicate a disorder of the heart valves. If there is any indication of heart enlargement, the doctor may try to confirm it by tapping the chest area around the heart. However, confirmation by imaging techniques is often employed.

THE RESPIRATORY SYSTEM

An examination of the respiratory system starts with an inspection of your chest, with special attention to symmetry, movement, and the degree of expansion. The doctor will also note the rate and nature of your breathing – whether it is smooth and easy, deep and labored, or short and painful.

Your doctor may also feel the central notch between your collarbones to ensure that your windpipe is lying centrally and is not deviated to one side. Deviation may be caused by a partially collapsed or shrunken lung, which can be a

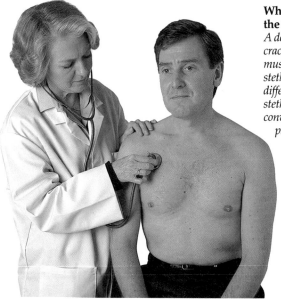

**What does
the doctor hear?**
*A doctor may hear
crackles, squeaks, or
musical notes through the
stethoscope as a result of
different disorders. The
stethoscope provides a
convenient substitute for
placing an ear to the
patient's body.*

Listening to the chest

Listening to your chest is one of the doctor's most valuable indicators of the state of your lungs. Breathing sounds are produced by the movement of air through the bronchi (the largest of the air passages). The character of these sounds is determined by the state of the surrounding lungs. Solid tissue conducts sound better, so both your breath and your voice are heard more clearly if you have lost any of the normal spongy consistency of your lungs.

Certain diseases cause additional sounds, such as wheezes, crackles, and various musical notes of different pitches. These sounds can indicate spasm of the bronchi, which occurs with bronchitis and asthma, or fluid in the air sacs, which occurs with pneumonia. Rubbing together of the layers of the lung lining, which is associated with pleurisy, causes the doctor to hear a characteristic creaking sound.

THE STETHOSCOPE

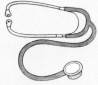

Symbol of the medical profession, the stethoscope is a pair of hollow plastic or rubber tubes connecting a piece that goes to the chest to a pair of earpieces. The chest piece is usually double-sided, with a bell-shaped end on one side and a diaphragm on the other. The bell is used to listen for low-pitched sounds and murmurs and the diaphragm for high-pitched ones. A stethoscope allows the doctor to use both ears at once (which increases sensitivity) and place the chest piece exactly where required (which allows greater precision).

cause of breathlessness at rest. The doctor may also ensure that expansion of your chest is the same on both sides by placing his or her hands symmetrically on either side of it and asking you to breathe deeply several times.

Percussion

A healthy chest is partly air-filled and resonant, making percussion an important element in a complete physical examination.

Fluid in the space between the lungs and the chest wall (the pleural space) causes a dull note when the doctor taps it, as does any solidification of the lung that occurs in certain conditions such as pneumonia. However, if the pleural space is filled with air, the percussion note will be highly resonant. The doctor may also place the sides of his or her hands firmly against your chest while you count out loud so he or she can feel the vibrations.

Peak flow meter
This device measures the maximum flow rate of air during expiration. The rate is reduced in certain respiratory disorders such as asthma.

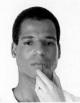

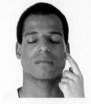
THE NERVOUS SYSTEM

The nervous system collects information about the body and its environment, analyzes it, and responds. If your medical history suggests a disorder of the nervous system, your doctor will want to assess the state of your intellectual functions, powers of concentration and attention, and memory.

Speech and motor ability

Your speech is also of interest to the doctor, who will want to determine whether there is any physical disorder affecting your speech apparatus or any defect in your ability to use language. Problems such as the inability to recall the names of common objects, or difficulties in understanding or expressing language, can indicate damage to different areas of the brain.

The doctor will also check your motor ability, or power of movement, by asking you to grip both of his or her hands and push your arms and legs against resistance in various directions. Any differences in the muscle power of the two sides of your body are noted.

You may also be asked to demonstrate your ability to walk normally. This is

Doctor restrains arm

Testing motor ability
You will be asked to push or pull against resistance in various directions. The doctor will note any difference in muscle power between the two sides of your body.

Patient attempts to flex arm at elbow

possible only if several different, integrated parts of your nervous system are working correctly. Any defect in this highly complex system is likely to be reflected in abnormality of gait.

Sensory information

The nerves that carry sensory information – for touch, pain, temperature, vibration, and position sense – from your body to your brain are checked next. With your eyes closed, the doctor stimulates certain skin areas by pricking your skin gently, brushing it lightly with cotton, and holding a vibrating tuning fork to the skin over a bony surface.

The doctor again compares one side of your body to the other. If one side only is able to respond to the stimulus, it is likely that there is a problem with one side of the nervous system.

Testing reflexes

The doctor will also test the deep tendon reflexes at your wrists, at the fronts and backs of your knees, and at your ankles. If the nerves from the spinal cord to the muscles (and those from the muscles to the cord) are functioning correctly, a sudden stretching of a muscle tendon by striking it with a rubber hammer will cause the muscle to tighten.

This nerve circuit, known as the reflex arc, is normally under the strict control of impulses from the brain. If these controlling influences are removed, which occurs with brain damage from a stroke, the reflexes become much brisker than usual. However, if there is damage to the nerves running to or from the spinal cord, the reflex jerk is absent.

Another important reflex test is the plantar reflex. To test this, the doctor firmly strokes the sole of your foot with a blunt instrument and watches the direction in which your toes move. Normally, the toes curl downward; if they fan upward, this is a sign of damage to the motor nerve pathways in the spinal cord or brain and necessitates more testing.

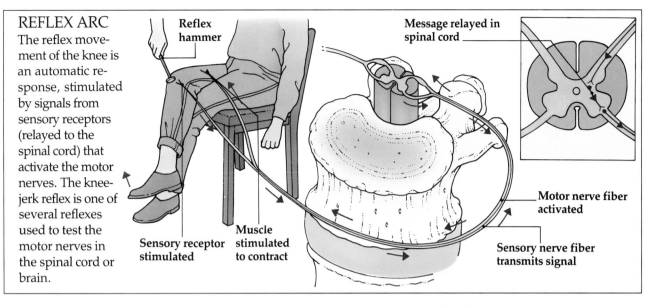

REFLEX ARC
The reflex movement of the knee is an automatic response, stimulated by signals from sensory receptors (relayed to the spinal cord) that activate the motor nerves. The knee-jerk reflex is one of several reflexes used to test the motor nerves in the spinal cord or brain.

Reflex hammer

Message relayed in spinal cord

Motor nerve fiber activated

Sensory nerve fiber transmits signal

Sensory receptor stimulated

Muscle stimulated to contract

THE LOCOMOTOR SYSTEM

This system encompasses your muscles, bones, and joints. The locomotor system is affected by any disorders of the nervous system that affect movement.

An examination of the locomotor system begins with a careful inspection of the joints. The doctor looks for any deformity or swelling and any discoloration or wasting of surrounding muscles. He or she will also check the range of motion in your hips, knees, and ankles.

Restriction of joint movement due to inflammation in the joint may be caused by a sprain of an external joint or of a joint cartilage, or by internal damage, such as cartilage and bone destruction caused by osteoarthritis, a torn ligament or cartilage, or a deformity from a condition such as rheumatoid arthritis.

THE LOWER BACK

The lower back is the site of many medical problems and the source of more pain than almost any other part of the body. The lumbar spine is affected by a variety of conditions, including misalignment of the joints, muscle strain, loss of bone strength, and osteoarthritis.

A prolapsed (herniated) disc
Most common of all is the tendency for the discs between the vertebrae to degenerate. When a disc breaks down, the pulpy interior is squeezed out (prolapses) and presses on a spinal nerve root, causing pain. This condition is often mistakenly called a "slipped" disc. Your doctor may test for a prolapsed disc by asking you to lie on your back, straighten your knee, and raise your leg. If the disc is prolapsed, it will press on the root of the sciatic nerve, causing pain and a limited range of motion.

Testing for a prolapsed disc
If the disc is prolapsed, you will be unable to lift your leg as far as normal when lying on your back without the onset of severe pain.

View of retina

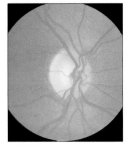

The ophthalmoscope
This device allows the doctor to see the retina at the back of the eye. With its small arteries and veins, the retina reflects the condition of the arteries and veins elsewhere in the body.

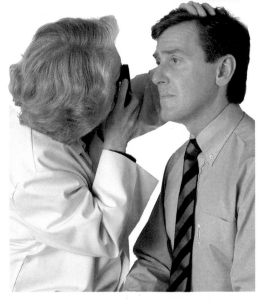

Urine test
Simple chemical tests can detect glucose, protein, or blood in urine. In the test shown here, a tablet added to a urine sample (right) produces a color change that indicates the glucose level (above).

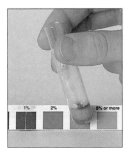

View of eardrum

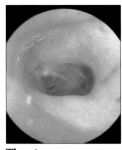

The otoscope
This is a simple instrument designed to provide illumination, and sometimes magnification, of the eardrum. The otoscope reveals any redness, inflammation, or perforation.

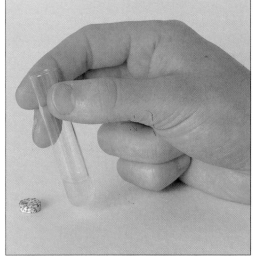

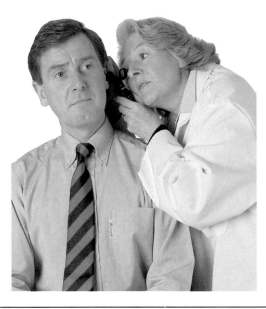

THE EYE

Your medical history may suggest a loss of vision that is unlikely to be correctable by glasses. Symptoms such as a partial loss of vision in one eye, the feeling of a black curtain coming across part of your visual field, a transient loss of vision, or the persistent loss of half the field of vision in both eyes suggest different problems to your doctor.

Many eye problems involve the external parts of the eye, such as the lids, cornea, and conjunctiva. Your doctor may want to examine these structures under magnification, which is achieved by the use of a hand lens.

THE URINARY SYSTEM

A history of urinary problems will prompt your doctor to feel your abdomen for any distention of your bladder. He or she will examine you to check for enlargement and tenderness of the kidneys. In men, a rectal examination to feel for enlargement of the prostate gland is usually also performed.

You may be asked to provide a specimen of urine, which may be examined in the doctor's office. In some cases, the specimen is sent directly to a laboratory for more sophisticated testing.

THE EAR

Hearing is tested, one ear at a time, by determining whether or not you are able to accurately hear whispered words or the ticking of a pocket watch in a quiet room. Some doctors use portable audiometers, which measure hearing loss for sounds of different pitches.

The external ear and the external auditory canal may also be checked for skin disorders. Your doctor can remove any excess earwax by syringing with warm water or by suction. Your eardrums may be examined with a special instrument called an otoscope.

CASE HISTORY
A PATIENT WITH A TREMOR

MARVIN SAW his family doctor several months ago because of a persistent trembling of his hands, which was getting progressively worse. The doctor initially thought that the trembling might not be a sign of any underlying disease and suggested waiting to see how things would evolve. When no improvement occurred during the following 2 weeks, however, the doctor suggested that Marvin make an appointment with a neurologist.

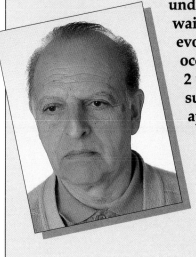

PERSONAL DETAILS
Name Marvin Hill
Age 59
Occupation Publisher
Family Marvin's father died several years ago of a heart attack. His mother is in relatively good health.

MEDICAL BACKGROUND
In addition to the tremor, Marvin complains of being easily fatigued and prone to backaches. He also has a tendency toward depression.

THE CONSULTATION
The neurologist takes a detailed medical history but can find little of relevance to a disorder of the nervous system. Marvin shows no signs of intellectual deterioration. His vision, hearing, taste, and sense of smell all appear to be normal, and there is no suggestion of any problem with sensation.

THE NEUROLOGIST'S IMPRESSION
During conversation, the neurologist notices some odd aspects in Marvin's manner, which suggests the diagnosis to her.

Marvin sits very still in his chair, bent forward, and speaks in a quiet, monotonous tone of voice. His face has a masklike lack of expression. The neurologist's suspicions lead her to investigate further.

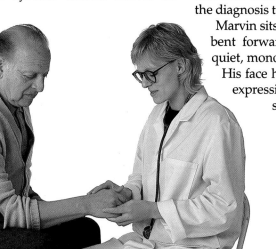

Investigating the tremor
When she examines Marvin's hand tremor, the neurologist notices it is present only when the hand is at rest – a characteristic sign of Parkinson's disease.

FURTHER INVESTIGATION
The neurologist inspects Marvin's hand tremor and finds it to be of a characteristic type, known as "pill-rolling," in which the pads of the thumb and forefinger move steadily and repetitively across one another. The forearm, too, shows a constant slight rotatory movement.

When he is asked to stand up, Marvin is a little bent forward and slightly rigid in both his neck and trunk. In addition, his limbs are bent and his muscles are stiff. All of his movements are slow.

The neurologist asks Marvin to take a few steps. His gait is slow and the steps are short and shuffling. His arms remain bent and do not swing. Once Marvin begins walking, he seems to have difficulty stopping. When he does stop, the specialist gently pushes him to one side, and Marvin totters until he finally comes to rest against the wall.

THE DIAGNOSIS
The neurologist feels confident in reaching a diagnosis of PARKINSON'S DISEASE, a disorder of part of the brain involved in the control of body movements. This is typical of a diagnosis that can be made in the doctor's office from observing a few classic signs. These signs include trembling, a masklike face, rigidity, and slowness. A shuffling, unbalanced walk is another typical sign; this was the reason that the neurologist asked Marvin to walk for her. Marvin's gait and posture confirmed the doctor's suspicions.

THE TREATMENT
The doctor prescribes a course of antiparkinsonism drugs. Although there is no cure for Parkinson's disease, drug treatment can give much relief from the illness and offers an improved quality of life.

CHAPTER THREE

X-RAYS AND SCANS

THE DISCOVERY of X-rays by Wilhelm Conrad Roentgen in 1895 revolutionized medical diagnosis by allowing doctors to see organs and structures inside the living body. Before this time, the only way the validity of a diagnosis for an internal disorder could be confirmed was to perform an operation or to wait and conduct an autopsy after the patient had died. Conventional X-rays have played an invaluable role in medicine for nearly a century, but their usefulness has proved to be limited. The images produced by X-rays are basically flat shadow photographs, even with the refinement of introducing contrast media into the body to enhance the imaging capability. In addition, exposing the patient to X-rays carries some risk (although a small one), of damaging body cells. Further, some types of contrast X-ray imaging can be uncomfortable, or the contrast medium may induce an allergic reaction. Today, technology is moving fast to overcome these limitations, and a new era in diagnostic imaging of the body is beginning. In many circumstances radiation-based techniques have been superseded by imaging methods that do not rely on radiation, which makes them completely safe for the patient. In ultrasound scanning

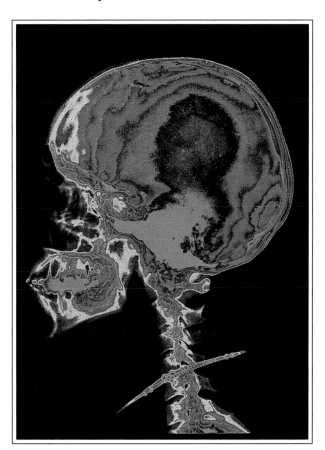

and Doppler scanning, for instance, the production of images is based on the detection of echoes that are returned from sound waves passed into the body. And, in an exciting new technique called magnetic resonance imaging (MRI), powerful magnets and radio waves provide the technical basis for the production of images.

X-ray imaging was transformed in the 1970s with the development of computed tomography (CT) scanning. This technique combines the use of multiple X-ray beams and detectors with a powerful computer to create cross-sectional and even three-dimensional images of body structures, providing doctors with highly detailed information. Computers are also used to create the cross-sectional images characteristic of ultrasound scanning and magnetic resonance imaging; they can also be used to enhance with color the images produced by most scans. Finally, computers have extended the capabilities of radionuclide scanning, a technique based on detection of radioactivity from substances introduced into body tissues. One refinement of radionuclide scanning is positron emission tomography (PET) scanning, which produces images that reflect the function of tissues – and their structure too.

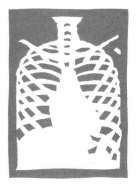

X-RAY IMAGING

DESPITE THE ADVENT of many new imaging techniques, X-rays are still a widely used and valuable means of seeing inside the body. The capabilities of X-ray imaging were limited at first, showing only dense body structures (such as bones) with any clarity. The development of contrast media extended the uses of X-rays by allowing the imaging of hollow and fluid-filled areas. More recently, computers have opened up new vistas for X-ray imaging.

In November 1895, Wilhelm Conrad Roentgen, professor of physics at the University of Würzburg, Germany, was experimenting with the flow of electricity through a vacuum tube. The electrical apparatus he was using was completely surrounded by black, light-proof cardboard. Yet, when Roentgen switched on the current, he became aware of a faint glimmer coming from a fluorescent screen lying on a nearby table. When he repeatedly switched the current on and off, the glow on the screen appeared and disappeared correspondingly.

During the following weeks, Roentgen was completely absorbed in investigating these mysterious rays that could penetrate matter. His most spectacular discovery occurred when he placed his hand in the path of the rays and saw the shadow of each of his bones appear on the fluorescent screen.

Roentgen had no idea of the nature of these new rays. Because "X" represents the unknown in algebra, he called them X-rays. The discovery was announced in December 1895 and rapidly became an important aid to medical diagnosis.

X-RAYS IN DIAGNOSIS

X-rays are a form of invisible electromagnetic radiation of short wavelength; they are closely related to both radio waves and light waves.

Doctors know to what extent each of the body's tissues absorbs X-rays. The less dense a substance is, the greater the ability of X-rays to pass through it. In the body, soft tissues – such as skin, fat, muscle, and blood – are more transparent to X-rays than hard, dense substances such as bone. Thus, when a beam of X-rays is directed at a part of the body – a leg, for example – X-rays pass easily through the soft tissues but do not penetrate the bone, which casts a shadow. Because X-rays blacken photographic film, the shadow of the bone appears as a white area; the soft tissues are represented on the film as dark gray.

Having an X-ray picture taken
Your position during the examination is carefully selected to obtain the best possible view of the part being examined. The X-ray technician will tell you exactly how to sit, stand, or lie. Because X-rays diverge as they leave the X-ray tube, it is important that the body part being X-rayed be placed as close as possible to the cassette containing the film. Otherwise, the image will be enlarged and details will be less clear. In most cases, the cassette is placed in contact with the area being X-rayed.

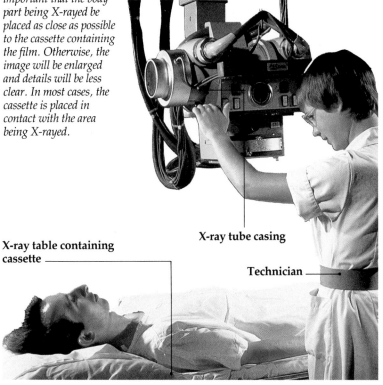

X-ray tube casing

X-ray table containing cassette

Technician

HOW X-RAYS ARE PRODUCED

X-rays are produced using electric power in a device called an X-ray tube, which contains an electron source (the cathode) and a nearby thick tungsten disc (the anode). When a high positive voltage is applied to the anode, the negatively charged electrons are strongly attracted to it; as they strike, X-rays are given off. The higher the voltage, the more energetic are the X-rays produced. The X-rays travel in straight lines, radiating outward from the target, and emerge as an X-ray beam from a small aperture in the lead casing that surrounds the X-ray tube.

The beam is focused on a part of the body placed against an X-ray cassette. When the film is processed, the body parts that allowed few X-rays to pass through appear white; those that transmitted many rays appear black. An identical image can also be produced on a fluorescent screen instead of on film. Today's X-ray equipment minimizes radiation exposure.

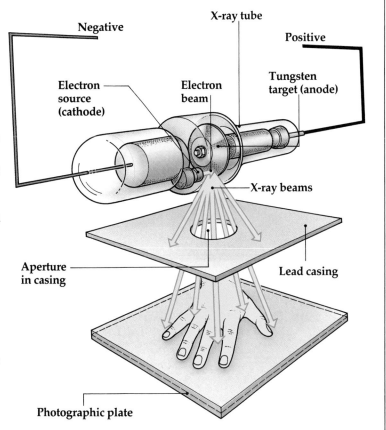

When are X-rays used?

X-rays give a photographic image of part of the body. This image may confirm or rule out the doctor's diagnosis, usually after other tests, such as blood or urine tests, have been performed.

The simplest type of X-ray examination is a single "snapshot" image. These plain X-ray pictures are an excellent means of showing bone and dense areas in the body, such as tumors, and are commonly used for examining the chest, skull, spine, and other parts of the skeleton. Hollow or fluid-filled organs do not show up well on plain X-rays but they, too, can be visualized using dyes and other contrast techniques (see CONTRAST X-RAY IMAGING on page 44). In many cases, plain X-rays and contrast techniques are being replaced by computed tomography (CT) scanning, which produces cross-sectional images of the body while exposing the patient to less radiation (see CT SCANNING on page 48).

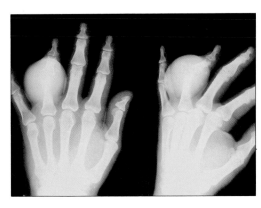

X-rays of a hand
These two color-enhanced X-rays of a hand show severe, gouty arthritis. The large, bright area around the middle joint of the ring finger is the result of the deposition of uric acid crystals and the consequent inflammation and swelling of the joint – a feature that is characteristic of gout.

PLAIN X-RAY EXAMINATIONS

When you arrive for an X-ray, the X-ray technician or radiologist will explain the procedure and will position you in contact with a cassette containing the X-ray film. You will be asked to remain very still during the period of exposure (which usually lasts less than a second), since any movement produces a blurred image that is difficult to interpret.

When all is ready – you are in the correct position, the film is in place, and the machine has been set to the right exposure – the technician moves briefly behind a protective screen (from which he or she can still see and talk to you) and presses the exposure button. You will not feel any sensation; X-rays are painless. The technician is screened to avoid being exposed to the radiation. A dose that is safe for you would, if repeated for the technician many times every day, eventually reach a dangerous level.

Taking the pictures

Several X-ray pictures are usually taken from different angles to get as complete a view as possible of the area in question. The technician will alter your position and that of the equipment as required between "takes." Sometimes it is necessary to support or even immobilize the part of the body being X-rayed. As soon as the pictures are taken, the films are passed into an automatic developing machine and are developed, fixed, and dried within a few minutes. If there is reason for urgency, the films are examined immediately by a radiologist. However, in most cases, the radiologist reviews your films later in his or her office, writes a formal report, and discusses the results with your doctor.

Risk of damage from X-rays
X-rays carry a small risk of producing damage to living tissues, which can lead to cancer. The risk can be expressed statistically in terms of the average number of examinations that would need to be carried out in a population to cause one cancer death. The chart below gives an idea of how small the risks are, and the comparative risks of different examinations.

RELATIVE RISKS OF X-RAYS

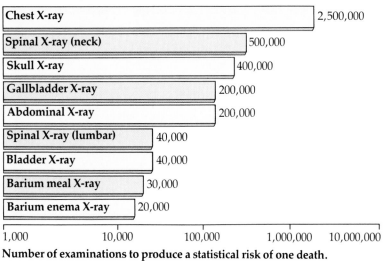

X-ray type	Number
Chest X-ray	2,500,000
Spinal X-ray (neck)	500,000
Skull X-ray	400,000
Gallbladder X-ray	200,000
Abdominal X-ray	200,000
Spinal X-ray (lumbar)	40,000
Bladder X-ray	40,000
Barium meal X-ray	30,000
Barium enema X-ray	20,000

1,000   10,000   100,000   1,000,000   10,000,000

Number of examinations to produce a statistical risk of one death.

ASK YOUR DOCTOR
X-RAYS

Q **I have had two spinal X-rays in the last 6 months because of my persistent back pain. Could exposure to all this radiation be dangerous?**

A Modern X-ray equipment and techniques are designed to produce high-quality pictures at the lowest possible radiation dose. All X-ray examinations carry a small risk of damaging living tissue. However, the benefits from obtaining a correct diagnosis and appropriate treatment using X-rays counterbalance the risk of exposure. The radiation dosage you have recently received from X-rays carries less risk than that of smoking a single pack of cigarettes.

Q **My son recently hurt his wrist in a fall off his skateboard and was told that the X-ray showed no fracture. However, we were advised that he should come back for another X-ray if the pain persisted. Why?**

A Fractures of the wrist bones, such as the scaphoid bone, may be impossible to detect on an X-ray taken soon after the fracture. However, fractures may become obvious later due to changes in the bone as it heals.

Q **I recently went to my doctor about a lump in my breast and she suggested I have a mammogram. Are there any risks from this procedure that I should consider?**

A A mammogram is an X-ray of the breast. The procedure is painless, and the dose of radiation is extremely small, so the risk of any damage to the breast tissue is negligible. In addition, the risk from the X-ray is outweighed by the benefit of early cancer detection, which gives the best chance of a cure.

CASE HISTORY
A BREATHLESS SMOKER

JIM'S BREATHING problems had been getting worse for several months. At first, the attacks of breathlessness occurred only when he exerted himself while walking around old buildings preparing estimates. But then Jim found himself gasping for air at rest. Even cutting down on his smoking didn't seem to help much. Faced with having to give up his demolition business, he decided to see his doctor.

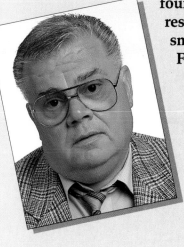

PERSONAL DETAILS
Name Jim O'Conner
Age 55
Occupation Demolition contractor
Family Mother suffers from mild heart failure.

MEDICAL BACKGROUND
Jim has been troubled for years by a persistent dry cough, which he attributes to his smoking.

THE CONSULTATION
Jim complains that he is suffering severe shortness of breath. During conversation with his doctor, he admits that his attacks of breathlessness first started years ago; he has long since given up heavy work because of them. The doctor discovers that, about 10 years ago, Jim's demolition work included stripping asbestos insulation from pipes.

When the doctor listens to the lower part of Jim's chest, she hears loud crackling noises toward the end of each inhalation.

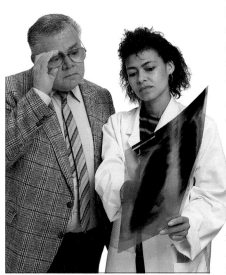

Chest X-ray
Jim's doctor orders a chest X-ray, which shows severe fibrosis (scar tissue formation) in the lungs. In the lower portion of Jim's lungs, the fibrosis is so advanced that it obscures the outline of the heart, causing a shaggy appearance.

THE DOCTOR'S IMPRESSION
Jim clearly has early respiratory failure due to a major lung disorder. The doctor suspects Jim's problems are related to his history of asbestos exposure and she orders a chest X-ray. Jim goes for the X-ray the next morning and the results are returned to the doctor in a few hours.

THE X-RAY FINDINGS
The X-rays confirm the doctor's suspicions. The films show irregular lines of shadowing in the lower zones of Jim's lungs, with a suggestion of honeycombing – an appearance indicating fibrosis (thickening and scarring) of the lung tissues. The X-rays also show marked thickening of the pleura (membranes that line the lungs) and a suggestion of fluid between the two layers of pleura.

THE DIAGNOSIS
From the X-ray findings and Jim's occupational history, the doctor reaches a diagnosis of ASBESTOSIS. As a result of long-term, persistent irritation by the asbestos fibers, Jim's lungs have been heavily invaded by a delicate collagen scar tissue. The area of his lungs that is available for oxygen transfer to the blood has been severely reduced. Jim's lungs are also severely restricted in their ability to expand because of the scarring. These two factors account for his severe breathlessness.

THE OUTLOOK
The damage to Jim's lungs is permanent, though he may benefit from oxygen therapy at some stage. But what seriously concerns the doctor is that Jim still smokes. Told that smoking and asbestosis give him a 50 percent chance of acquiring lung cancer, Jim quits smoking. After about 6 weeks he is able to move around more comfortably.

WHAT CAN X-RAYS SHOW?

The X-ray image, or radiograph, is a shadow picture of the shape and density of the parts of the body under examination. This makes X-rays of greatest use in diagnosing diseases and disorders that actually alter the structure of the body. The abnormalities in some X-ray images are subtle and may be apparent only to a radiologist – a doctor specializing in X-ray interpretation. In other X-ray pictures, the changes are so dramatic they are obvious to the untrained observer. The X-ray images below show conditions that range from the obvious, such

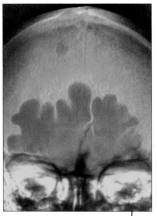

X-ray of the skull
The color-enhanced view of the skull above shows inflammation of the paranasal sinuses (the air spaces above the eye sockets), which appear orange here.

Dental X-ray
X-rays are invaluable to check for cavities and other abnormalities. The X-ray picture below shows fillings in several back teeth. The root tips of the top two canine teeth were removed and filled to treat an abscess.

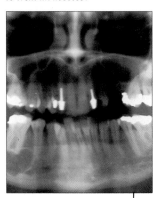

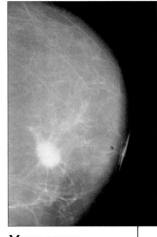

Mammogram
X-rays of the breast can show breast cancer at an early stage, when it is often completely curable. The white area on the mammogram above indicates early breast cancer.

Chest X-ray
Cancer in both lungs is evident in the color-enhanced image below. The cancerous areas appear on the image as distinct orange shadows. The heart is at the lower center, projecting to the right of the X-ray.

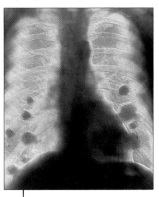

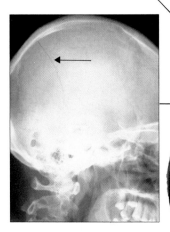

Skull X-ray (side view)
A hairline skull fracture can be seen as a fine line toward the back of the skull. An X-ray is the only means of detecting such delicate fractures of the skull.

as the white, cancerous area on the mammogram, to the subtle. An arrow has been added to the image of one skull X-ray to help you visualize the hairline fracture. Bones are much denser than other body tissues, so both healthy bone and abnormalities such as fractures are usually easy to see. Healthy lungs appear almost transparent, but denser areas in the lungs, such as patches of solidification caused by pneumonia, show up clearly. Solid organs, such as the kidneys and the liver, cast faint shadows on the X-ray film.

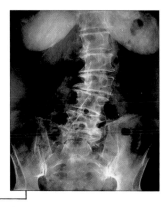

Pelvic X-ray
The hip joints shown in the X-ray below are severely crippled by rheumatoid arthritis. This X-ray was taken before an operation to replace the hip joints with artificial components. The drawing superimposed on the image shows where the new parts will be placed.

X-ray of lower leg
The color-enhanced X-ray below clearly shows a fracture of the tibia, the larger of the two bones in the lower leg.

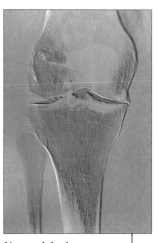

Spinal X-ray
The color-enhanced X-ray above shows curvature of the spine as well as narrowed spaces between the vertebrae (spinal bones) and bony outgrowths, which can be seen to the left of the lower five vertebrae.

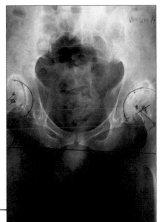

X-ray of the knee
Arthritis has affected the knee joint, causing the joint space to become extremely narrow. The X-ray is color-enhanced.

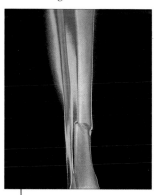

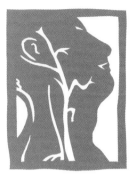

CONTRAST X-RAY IMAGING

BONES AND LUNGS show up well on plain X-rays, but most other body organs require enhancement. Hollow or fluid-filled body parts, such as blood vessels, the urinary tract, and the digestive tract, can be shown on an X-ray film if they are first filled with contrast media – solutions of substances that are opaque to X-rays.

The technique of contrast X-ray imaging can be applied to a large number of body organs and tissues (though, in some cases, it has been supplanted by new imaging methods). Four of the most commonly used contrast examinations are discussed here. Other contrast procedures, including myelography (examination of the spinal cord), hysterosalpingography (the uterus and fallopian tubes), and cholecystography (the gallbladder), are discussed in the A–Z OF MEDICAL TESTS on pages 128 to 141.

BARIUM X-RAY EXAMINATIONS

Barium examinations are used to investigate diseases or abnormalities in any part of the digestive tract, from the esophagus to the rectum. Before X-ray pictures are taken, a suspension of barium sulfate and water is passed into the area to be examined by swallowing it or introducing it into the body through a tube. Barium is a metallic element that is im-

TYPES OF BARIUM X-RAY EXAMINATION

Barium swallow, meal, and follow-through
You are not permitted to eat or drink for 6 to 9 hours before the examination, which investigates the esophagus, stomach, duodenum, and small intestine. If your swallowing mechanism is being tested (left), you will be given bread or a cookie soaked in barium. A series of X-ray pictures is then taken.

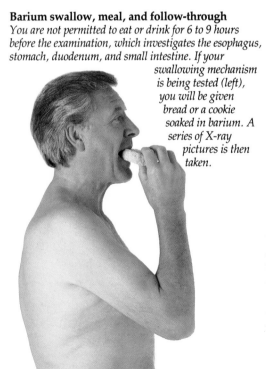

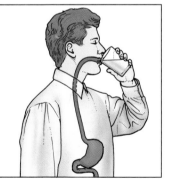

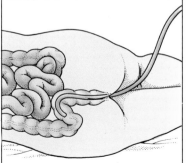

Barium small-bowel series
Food and liquids are not permitted for 9 hours before examination. You will be asked to swallow a glass of barium mixed with flavored liquid. Films are made at 15-minute intervals and again at hourly intervals. When a film shows barium has reached the colon, the radiologist examines the last portion of the small intestine by applying gentle pressure to the right lower portion of your abdominal wall while looking at the image on a screen.

Barium enema
To get a clear view of any abnormalities, the bowel must be as clean and empty as possible. You are asked not to eat or drink for 9 hours before the enema. At the examination, a tube is introduced into the rectum and barium is passed through it. With an air-contrast barium enema, barium is placed into the colon and then air is pumped into the colon. This technique puts the lining of the colon into contrast, permitting much better diagnosis of polyps and tumors.

pervious to X-rays, so it provides an image of the digestive tract on X-ray film.

Barium X-rays are useful in revealing narrowing of the esophagus, swallowing disorders, hiatal hernia, stomach polyps and tumors, ulcers of the stomach and duodenum, certain intestinal disorders such as diverticular disease, and tumors or polyps in the colon. You may be advised to have a barium examination before or after other investigations such as ENDOSCOPY (see page 68) if you are suffering from difficulty swallowing, stomach pains, inexplicable weight loss, a recent change in bowel habits, persistent diarrhea, or rectal bleeding.

Having a barium X-ray examination

Barium X-ray examinations are performed in the hospital as an outpatient procedure. No anesthetic is required. A fluorescent screen on which a moving image appears allows the radiologist to follow the progress of the barium through the digestive tract while observing any abnormalities outlined by the barium. Permanent records of the examination are provided by X-ray photographs or video recordings.

A barium swallow and a barium meal take about 15 minutes. In a barium small-bowel series, multiple X-rays are taken at intervals as the barium progresses through the small intestine. The examination is usually completed in 2 hours but, in some patients, may take up to 5 hours. A barium enema examination lasts about 20 to 25 minutes.

Barium liquid becomes firmer as it dries out in the large intestine, so you may become constipated after a barium examination. Make sure you drink at least 8 glasses of water daily for several days after the test and eat plenty of fiber-rich foods. If necessary, your doctor may recommend a laxative. For a few days after the examination, your stools will be white or pink, depending upon the color of the barium suspension used.

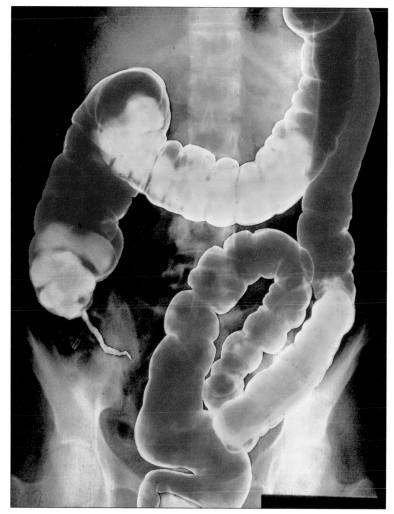

ANGIOGRAPHY

Angiography is a contrast technique that enables the doctor to see arteries and veins on an X-ray picture.

When is angiography used?

Angiography is used less frequently today in the early stages of investigation than it was in the past because other procedures such as CT SCANNING (see page 48), MAGNETIC RESONANCE IMAGING (see page 54), and DOPPLER SCANNING (see page 65) can give much the same information with less risk and discomfort to the patient. However, if surgery is being considered by the doctor and patient, an angiogram is still performed in many cases to give a clear, precise picture of the blood vessels.

Barium X-ray
This color-enhanced X-ray, taken after a barium enema, shows the large intestine. The diagram below shows the part of the body that has been imaged.

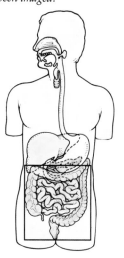

Angiography can reveal dangerous narrowing or other abnormalities of the carotid arteries and their branches, the vessels that supply blood to the brain. An operation on these vessels is occasionally performed to avoid a stroke. Angiography can also reveal the site of an aneurysm (a potentially dangerous weakening and ballooning of an artery) or tumor in the brain.

Another important application of angiography is in the investigation of coronary heart disease. It is used to identify areas of narrowing or blockage of the arteries that supply the heart muscle, allowing treatment to be planned accurately. When it is used for this purpose, angiography is often combined with CARDIAC CATHETERIZATION (see page 130).

Angiography is also used for investigating tumors, and diseases of the aorta (the largest artery), the leg arteries, and the arteries supplying the kidneys.

Having an angiogram

Before X-ray pictures are taken, contrast medium is injected into the vessel being investigated. For a carotid angiogram, this is usually achieved by inserting a catheter (narrow tube) into an artery in the groin; for a coronary angiogram, the catheter is often inserted into an artery at the front of the elbow.

First, a small injection of a local anesthetic is given into the tissues surrounding the artery. This procedure is almost painless and allows the doctor to slide a needle into the artery with the least possible discomfort to you. A long, thin wire with a smooth, rounded tip is then threaded through the needle and guided, under X-ray control, into the artery to be examined. When the wire is in place, the needle is removed, and the catheter is slipped over the wire and guided along until its tip is in the correct position. The wire is removed and contrast medium is injected into the catheter. During the injection, you may have a sensation of warmth lasting a few seconds; the feeling is often more pronounced in the area being examined.

The radiologist studies the flow of the dye along the arteries by watching the image on a screen or by taking a rapid sequence of X-ray pictures.

ANGIOGRAPHIC IMAGING

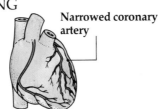

Narrowed coronary artery

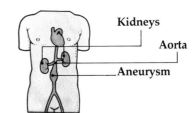

Kidneys

Aorta

Aneurysm

Angiogram
In this color-enhanced angiogram, the left coronary artery is shown to be severely narrowed. The narrowing, caused by atherosclerosis (the formation of fatty deposits on artery walls), restricts blood supply and deprives the heart muscle of oxygen. If a blood clot completely blocks the vessel, the section of heart muscle it supplies will die – an event known as a heart attack.

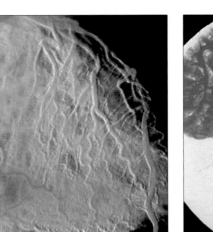

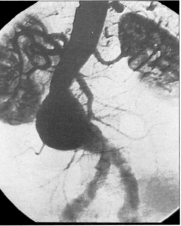

Digital subtraction angiogram
In this technique, an X-ray picture taken before the injection of contrast medium is subtracted electronically from an X-ray of the same area taken after the injection of the contrast medium. The result is a clear outline of the blood vessels. Shown in this example is an abdominal aneurysm (balloonlike swelling) on the largest artery, the aorta.

PYELOGRAPHY

This procedure is performed to obtain X-ray pictures of the urinary system. Pyelography involves the introduction of an iodine-based contrast medium into the kidneys, ureters, and bladder.

Pyelography may be used to investigate recurrent urinary tract or kidney infections, or the cause of blood in the urine. It can reveal abnormalities, such as kidney tumors or stones or an obstruction, anywhere in the urinary system.

Undergoing pyelography

For intravenous pyelography you will be asked not to eat or drink for up to 12 hours before the examination. You also may be given a laxative.

During the examination, you lie down while X-ray pictures are taken of your abdomen. You are then given an injection of contrast medium into a vein in your arm, and more X-ray pictures are taken at 5-, 10-, and 30-minute intervals as the contrast medium passes from the blood into the kidneys and then down the ureters. When your bladder is filled, another X-ray picture is taken. You are asked to urinate; when you have emptied your bladder, an X-ray is taken to see how well the bladder has emptied.

Retrograde pyelography is performed by a urologist in a surgical suite; topical anesthesia and a sedative are required. A cystoscope (viewing tube) is passed into the bladder and a narrow tube is threaded through it and guided up a ureter to one of the kidneys. Contrast medium is then injected through the tube and X-ray pictures are taken.

What are the risks?

Pyelography is generally very safe. However, because iodine is a constituent of the contrast medium used in this procedure, pyelography is not performed on people who are sensitive to iodine. Retrograde pyelography may aggravate infection of the urinary system.

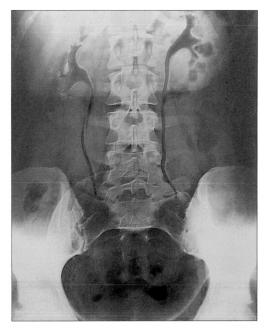

ERCP

Endoscopic retrograde cholangiopancreatography (ERCP) is a special contrast X-ray examination of the ducts that lead from the liver, gallbladder, and pancreas into the duodenum (the first part of the small intestine). A contrast medium is introduced into these ducts via an endoscope passed down your throat.

ERCP reveals abnormalities (such as gallstones) or irregularities in the ducts that are caused by disease processes such as inflammation, cirrhosis of the liver, or cancer.

You will be asked not to eat or drink for at least 8 hours before ERCP. An intravenous infusion is started before the examination, and you will be given a sedative by injection to make you feel sleepy, although you will remain conscious throughout the procedure. A topical anesthetic may be sprayed on your throat to reduce any discomfort caused by the endoscope.

After X-ray pictures have been taken, the endoscope is slowly removed. Your throat may be sore for a little while and you may feel the need to belch. You will not be allowed to eat or drink anything for several hours after the examination.

Intravenous pyelogram
The urine-collecting ducts of the kidneys and the ureters leading to the bladder are seen outlined in red in this color-enhanced pyelogram. The kidneys are functioning normally.

Having ERCP
An endoscope (a flexible viewing instrument) is passed down the back of the throat, through the esophagus and stomach, and into the duodenum. Once the endoscope is in the duodenum, you may be turned facedown. The doctor then passes a cannula (a tiny, flexible tube) via a side channel in the endoscope into the duct system. A contrast medium is injected and X-ray pictures are taken.

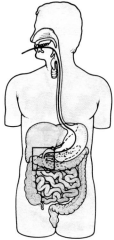

Endoscope   Contrast medium

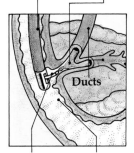

Cannula   Duodenum

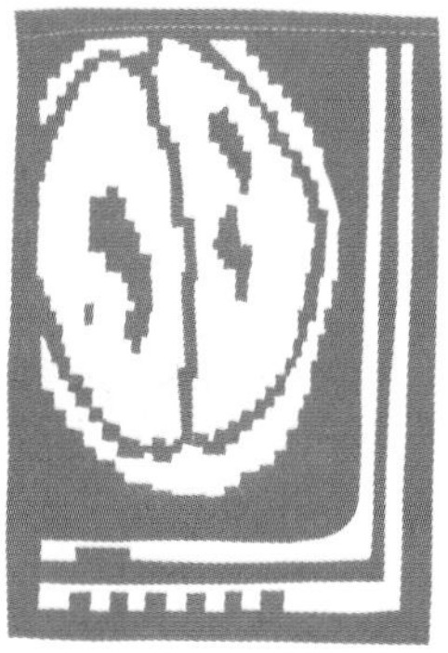

CT SCANNING

THE DEVELOPMENT of computed tomography (CT) scanning in the 1970s marked a breakthrough in medical diagnosis. The technique uses X-rays that are passed through the body at many angles in conjunction with a computer to produce cross-sectional images ("slices") through structures such as the head and abdomen.

A CT scanner is an X-ray machine with a difference. Instead of sending one X-ray beam through your body, the scanner sends a succession of very narrow beams at different angles. An array of detectors picks up the beams – which are weakened by differing amounts by the tissues they pass through – and sends signals to a computer. From the information provided, the computer can reconstruct a two-dimensional slice through the body, which is displayed on a TV screen.

CT images are more detailed than those produced by X-rays alone and can be manipulated using a computer so that tissues can be seen from different angles or even in three dimensions. In addition, CT scanning minimizes the amount of radiation exposure to the patient.

Having a CT scan
To have a CT scan, you lie on a sliding table that moves into the large circular opening of the CT machine (below). Each scan takes 2 to 5 seconds to perform. During the scan, low dosage X-ray beams are produced by a small X-ray source within the scanner, which rotates around you, and the radiation is picked up by detectors on the other side of the scanner (far right). With each pulse of radiation, the detectors produce electrical outputs that are stored in a computer.

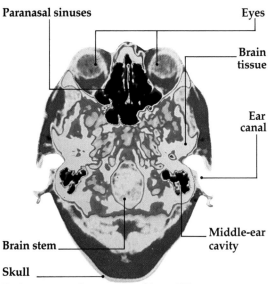

Paranasal sinuses · **Eyes** · **Brain tissue** · **Ear canal** · **Middle-ear cavity** · **Brain stem** · **Skull**

Brain cross section produced by a CT scan
From information stored during the scan, the computer is able to reconstruct an image of a cross section through the body, such as the color-enhanced slice through the brain (at the level of the eyes) shown above. The different colors correspond to tissues of varying densities. Several structures and cavities within the head can be seen on this CT scan.

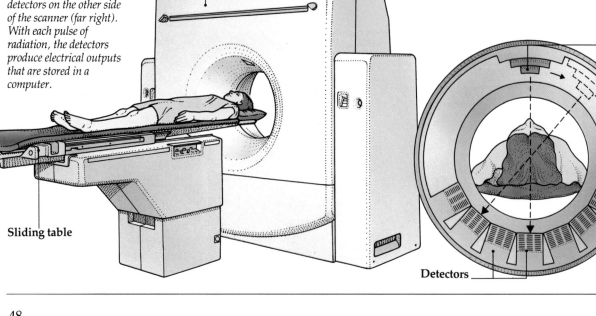

Scanner can be tilted to obtain different cross sections

X-ray source

Sliding table

Detectors

Abdominal scan
For an abdominal scan, the patient is moved farther into the scanning machine. The color-enhanced image at right shows a slice through the abdomen at a level just above the waist, revealing soft organs such as the liver and pancreas as well as the ribs and spine.

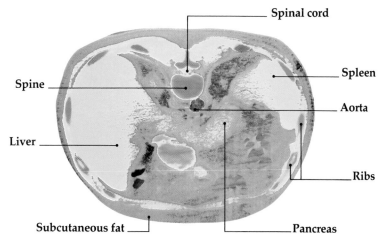

Spinal cord

Spine

Liver

Spleen

Aorta

Ribs

Subcutaneous fat

Pancreas

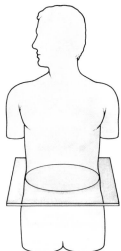

Site of cross section

DIAGNOSTIC USES

CT scanning was originally developed to look specifically at the brain, but its use has been extended to examine virtually every part of the body. The technique is especially valuable for investigating the brain for tumors, bleeding, aneurysms (balloonlike swellings on arteries), or injuries. It can be used to detect tumors and abscesses anywhere in the abdomen and to reveal damage to organs in cases of severe· injury. Lacerations of the spleen, kidney, or liver, which can occur in serious automobile accidents, can be seen immediately on a CT scan.

Preparing for the procedure
Before some CT scans, you may be given an injection of a contrast medium containing iodine that will clearly show certain blood vessels, organs, or abnormalities such as tumors. You will feel the minor discomfort of the needle prick and some warmth with the injection.

For an abdominal scan, you may be asked not to eat or drink anything for 12 hours except for a diluted barium solution that lines the bowel and makes it easier to see on the scan.

Having a CT scan
During the scan, you lie on a table with the part of your body to be examined within the circular opening of the scanner. You will not feel any sensation as the X-rays pass through you. Soon an image, viewed by the radiologist, appears on the screen attached to the console of the instrument.

You may feel the table on which you are lying move a little every few seconds as each image is obtained. The amount of time it takes to complete the examination will depend on how many exposures are made during each slice and on the number of angles required. It may also take the technician a little time to position you correctly and set up the machine.

INTERPRETATION

Ordinary X-rays can detect only several different levels of contrast among bones, soft tissues, and other internal organs. CT scans can detect hundreds of levels, bringing out details, especially of soft tissues, that are impossible to see with conventional X-rays. Body tissues that have differing densities, such as bone, fat, and muscle, are clearly delineated on the image produced by a CT scan.

The images produced in brain scans show the brain's ventricles (fluid-filled spaces) in particularly sharp definition. Abdominal CT scans reveal with ease some organs, such as the pancreas and the adrenal glands, that are not visible on ordinary X-ray pictures.

The findings of CT scans are highly accurate in most cases.

IS CT SCANNING SAFE?
In terms of radiation dosage, CT scans are safer than conventional X-rays. Many CT examinations would have to be performed to risk damaging the patient's cells or tissue.

The risk is greater if a scan is done in conjunction with a contrast medium, to which some people are allergic. Reactions to repeated contact with contrast media can be severe, so always tell your doctor if you have had a previous reaction. You should also tell your doctor if you have a history of kidney trouble, since the contrast medium in some cases damages diseased kidneys.

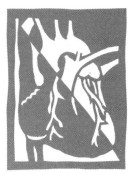

RADIONUCLIDE SCANNING

X-RAY TECHNIQUES use an external source of radiation that is passed through the body. In radionuclide scanning, however, a radioactive substance is introduced into the body and the radiation given off is detected by a special camera. Because tiny amounts of radiation are used, the procedure is considered very safe. In fact, the exposure to radiation during a radionuclide scan is usually less than that from a standard X-ray examination of the chest or skull.

Gamma camera
The radioactive substance inside your body gives off gamma rays that are detected by a gamma camera such as the one shown below. The gamma camera contains many sodium iodide crystals, which respond to gamma rays by emitting small flashes of light (scintillations). Detectors surrounding the crystal convert the flashes to electronic signals, which a computer converts to produce an image.

Radionuclide scanning, also known as scintigraphy, has been used as an imaging technique for more than 30 years. Terms like heart scan, bone scan, and thyroid scan generally refer to radionuclide scanning as opposed to other types of imaging techniques.

DIAGNOSTIC USES

When swallowed or injected into the body, different radioactive substances, known as radionuclides or radioisotopes, are taken up in greater quantities by some tissues than by others, making it possible to study specific organs.

Radioactive iodine, for example, concentrates in the thyroid gland. A higher or lower than normal concentration of iodine in the thyroid indicates overactivity or underactivity of the gland.

Radionuclide scanning can detect some diseases at an earlier stage than other imaging techniques because changes in the way an organ functions often occur before any structural changes take place. For example, bone infection stimulates blood flow and cell activity. This activity results in an increased radionuclide uptake in the bones before any changes in the structure of the bones can be seen on X-ray pictures.

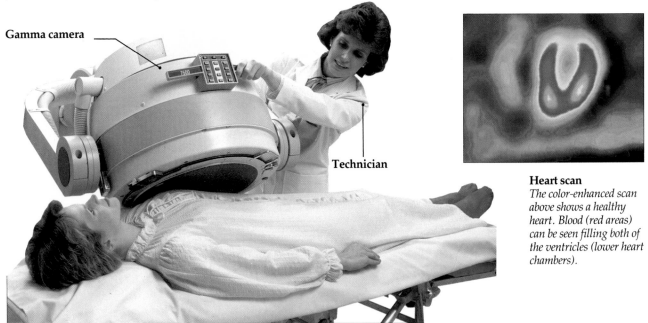

Gamma camera

Technician

Heart scan
The color-enhanced scan above shows a healthy heart. Blood (red areas) can be seen filling both of the ventricles (lower heart chambers).

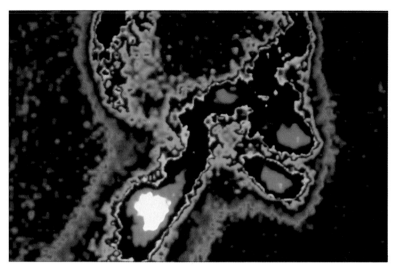

Radionuclide scanning is widely used for detecting small areas of tissue damage. After a heart attack, for instance, the extent of heart muscle damage can be assessed by using a substance that concentrates in damaged muscle cells but not in normal cells. Some radionuclides concentrate in tumors, making full body scanning a useful method of locating tumors and determining the extent of cancer spread.

Moving images can be used to study such functions as blood flow, emptying of the stomach, heart movements, the flow of urine through the kidneys, or the flow of bile through the liver.

How a scan works

After injection, the radionuclide travels to the target organ, where it emits gamma rays (like X-rays, only of shorter wavelength) that can be detected by a gamma camera. A computer analyzes the results and builds an image that can be displayed on a screen or in numerical form. A moving image can also be created by taking a series of pictures as the radionuclide passes through the body.

A specialized type of radionuclide scanning, known as single photon emission computed tomography (SPECT), enables cross-sectional images to be created by using a gamma camera that rotates around the patient. The principles are similar to those of computed tomog-

Bone scan
This color-enhanced scan shows cancer affecting the spinal bones in the neck. The radionuclide injected before the scan concentrates more strongly in cancerous bone than in normal bone and shows up as a white "hot spot" on the image.

raphy (CT) scanning (see page 48). Positron emission tomography (PET) scanning is a novel type of radionuclide scanning that is proving valuable in the study of depression, brain tumors, and heart conditions (see page 52).

SCANNING PROCEDURE

Radionuclide scanning causes little discomfort. For most scans, the radionuclide is injected into a vein in your arm; in some cases, you are asked to drink a radioactive solution. The scan may proceed immediately or you may have to wait for up to 4 hours. In some cases, you will need to return for more scans at intervals of days or weeks.

To have the scan, you will be asked to sit or lie down. The gamma camera is moved close to the part of your body being examined so that it can detect the radiation emitted from your body. You will feel nothing, but you may be asked to move into different positions. During the scan itself, you must remain still. The amount of time the procedure takes depends on the type of examination.

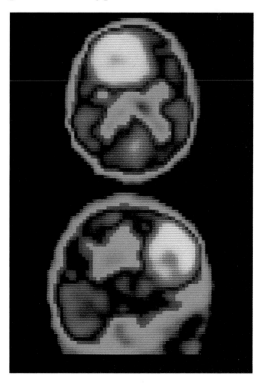

Brain scans
These two brain scans, which clearly show a large rounded tumor in the front of the brain, were taken by SPECT (single photon emission computed tomography). The upper image shows a horizontal "slice" through the head, and the lower image a vertical slice (the patient is facing to the right).

What are the risks?

Radionuclide scanning is a safe procedure. The radionuclides emit only a tiny amount of radiation compared to that used in X-ray examinations and they soon decay to harmless nonradioactive substances. Because the radionuclide is injected or taken by mouth, the procedure also avoids the risks of some other procedures such as cardiac catheterization. There is virtually no risk of an allergic reaction to radionuclides.

Interpretation

Once the scan is completed, the radiologist will discuss the result of the scan with you or with your doctor. Radionuclide scanning can provide vital information on a wide range of disorders affecting most parts of the body. The sensitivity of detection is high and, in many cases, the method can reveal abnormalities at an earlier stage than other tests, increasing the chances of a complete cure.

PET SCANNING

Positron emission tomography (PET) scanning is a special form of radionuclide scanning. It uses radioisotopes that have been specially manufactured so they will emit particles called positrons. The radioisotopes can be tagged on to a wide range of biologically important substances such as glucose or hormones. These radioactively tagged substances are injected into the blood or inhaled.

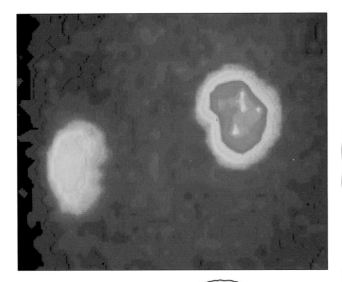

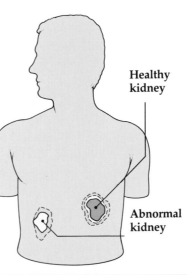

Kidney scan
This color-enhanced scan of the kidneys shows a healthy left kidney and a right kidney with a greatly reduced blood supply. More radionuclide is taken up by the healthy kidney, which appears bright red on the image, than by the abnormal kidney.

Healthy kidney

Abnormal kidney

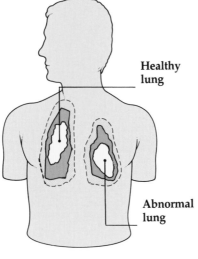

Lung scan
Radionuclide lung scanning helps in detecting disease by showing whether normal amounts of blood and oxygen are reaching the lungs. In this scan, the irregular uptake of radionuclide (yellow area) in the lung on the right indicates that it is receiving an insufficient blood supply.

Healthy lung

Abnormal lung

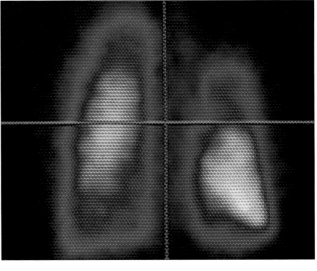

Having a PET scan
When you have a PET scan, you lie on a table that moves you into a large, doughnut-shaped device, which contains several stacked rings of detectors. You will have an injection just before the examination, have an infusion, or inhale a radioactive gas while you are within the scanner. The procedure is painless.

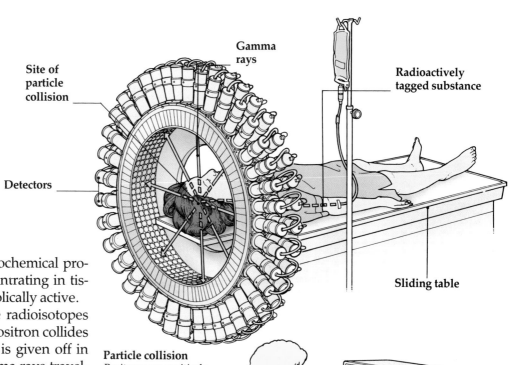

Site of particle collision

Gamma rays

Radioactively tagged substance

Detectors

Sliding table

They then take part in biochemical processes in the body, concentrating in tissues that are more metabolically active.

Within the tissues, the radioisotopes emit positrons. When a positron collides with an electron, energy is given off in the form of a pair of gamma rays traveling in opposite directions. By surrounding the patient with a ring of detectors linked to a computer, the point of origin of these rays can be calculated and an image plotted on a monitor. Because radioisotopes that emit positrons are very short-lived (some decay in a matter of minutes), the cyclotron that produces them must be located near the PET scanner. A cyclotron is a complex and expensive piece of equipment, restricting PET scanning to only a few medical centers.

Why is it done?

PET scanning is valuable because the images produced reflect the chemical and metabolic activity of the tissues under investigation. One of its principal uses has been to study the brain. It can detect tumors, locate the source of epileptic activity, and provide information about brain function in mental illnesses. PET scanning is also proving to be beneficial in the study of the heart. By revealing areas of decreased blood flow and cell activity in the heart muscle, this technique can help predict whether the heart muscle will recover after a heart attack has occurred.

Particle collision
Positrons are positively charged particles given off by some radioactive substances. When a positron collides with a negatively charged electron, the particles annihilate each other and two gamma rays are released (below).

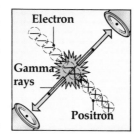

Electron

Gamma rays

Positron

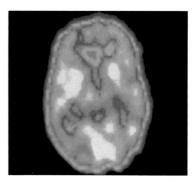

Building a picture
As the scanner detects the source of gamma rays given off from the patient's tissues, a picture of positron emission, and thus of the distribution of the radioactively tagged substance, can be constructed by a computer linked to the scanner (above). The image created on the screen is a cross section of the part of the body being examined, color coded according to the concentration of radioactivity.

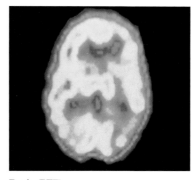

Brain PET scans
These PET scans were taken after injection of radioactively labeled glucose. In the brain of a person

suffering from depression (left), there is less uptake of glucose (green), indicating a lower level of brain activity, than in a healthy person's brain (right).

MAGNETIC RESONANCE IMAGING

MAGNETIC RESONANCE IMAGING (MRI) is a valuable diagnostic technique that has been used since the early 1980s. MRI provides high-quality, cross-sectional, or even three-dimensional, images of organs and structures within the body without using X-rays or other potentially harmful radiation. The technique is based on the use of a magnetic field and radio waves.

The MRI scanner was originally known as a nuclear magnetic resonance scanner. The word "nuclear" was dropped because it suggested that nuclear radiation was used in the procedure although, in fact, no nuclear radiation is involved.

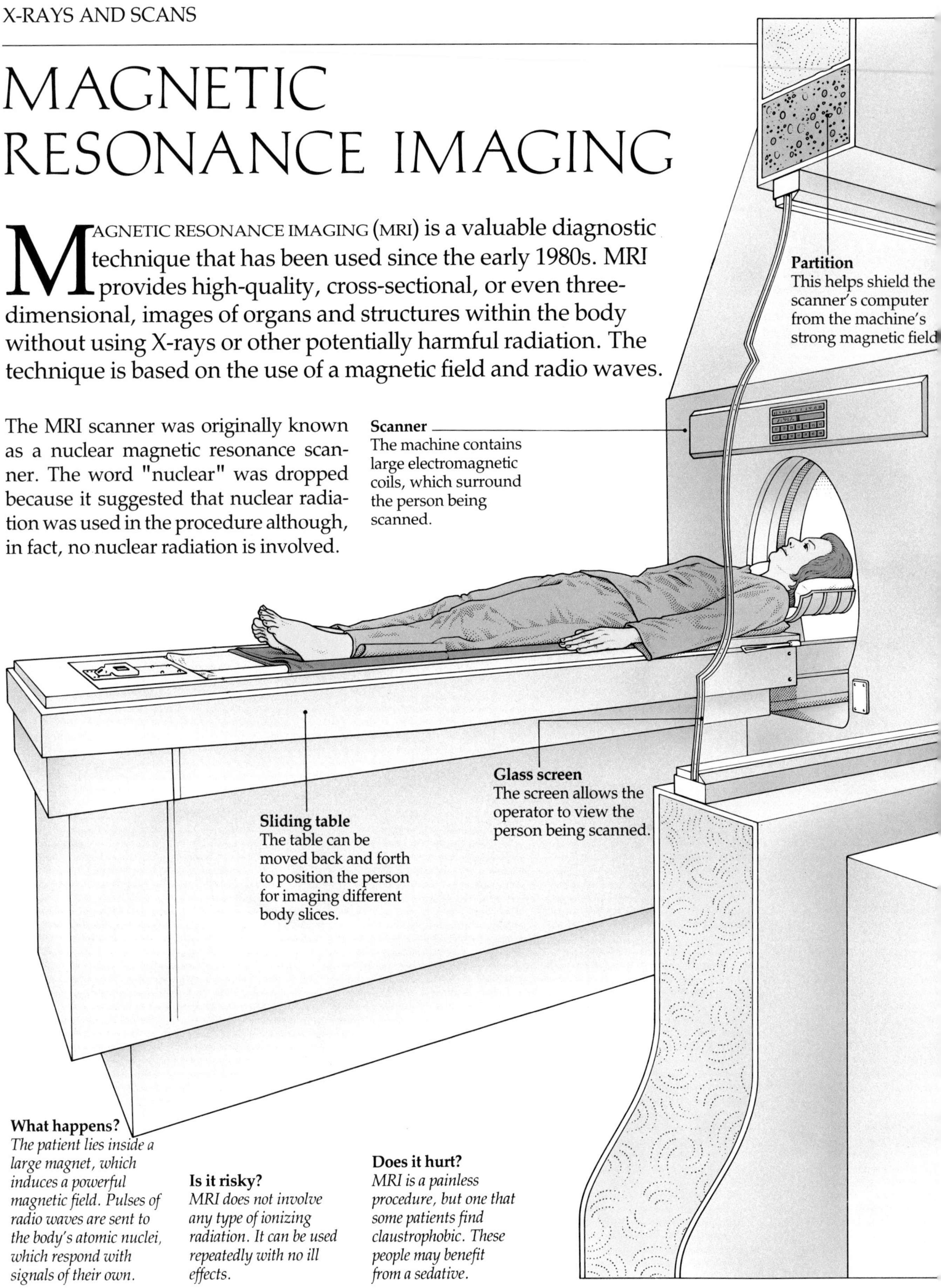

Partition
This helps shield the scanner's computer from the machine's strong magnetic field

Scanner
The machine contains large electromagnetic coils, which surround the person being scanned.

Glass screen
The screen allows the operator to view the person being scanned.

Sliding table
The table can be moved back and forth to position the person for imaging different body slices.

What happens?
The patient lies inside a large magnet, which induces a powerful magnetic field. Pulses of radio waves are sent to the body's atomic nuclei, which respond with signals of their own.

Is it risky?
MRI does not involve any type of ionizing radiation. It can be used repeatedly with no ill effects.

Does it hurt?
MRI is a painless procedure, but one that some patients find claustrophobic. These people may benefit from a sedative.

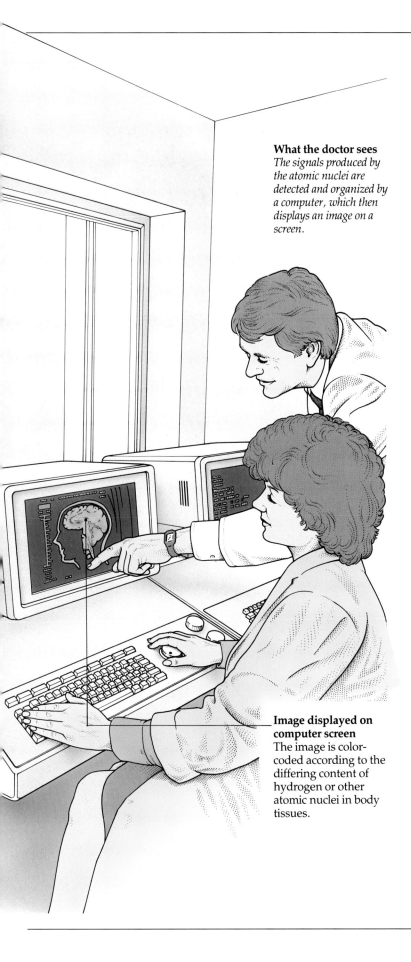

What the doctor sees
The signals produced by the atomic nuclei are detected and organized by a computer, which then displays an image on a screen.

Image displayed on computer screen
The image is color-coded according to the differing content of hydrogen or other atomic nuclei in body tissues.

MRI BRAIN SCAN

Skull

Cerebrum

Cerebellum

Brain stem

Upper spinal cord

Shown is a color-enhanced MRI scan of a vertical section through a person's head, highlighting the brain. The image clearly shows the convoluted surface of the cerebrum (main mass of the brain), the cerebellum at the back of the brain, the brain stem, and the top part of the spinal cord. The colors correspond to differing water contents in the tissues of the brain.

HOW MRI WORKS

The patient lies inside a huge, hollow, cylindrical magnet in which the body is exposed to a magnetic field 10,000 to 30,000 times more powerful than the earth's magnetic field. The nuclei of the body's atoms normally point randomly in different directions. In a magnetic field, however, they line up parallel to each other, like rows of tiny magnets. If the nuclei are knocked out of alignment by a strong pulse of radio waves, they produce detectable radio signals as they realign themselves.

Radio receiver coils in the machine detect these signals and a computer converts them into an image based on the

HOW DOES MRI WORK?

During an MRI scan, you lie surrounded by the coils of a powerful, supercooled electromagnet. A second electromagnetic coil, capable of delivering pulses of radio-frequency energy, surrounds the part of your body to be imaged.

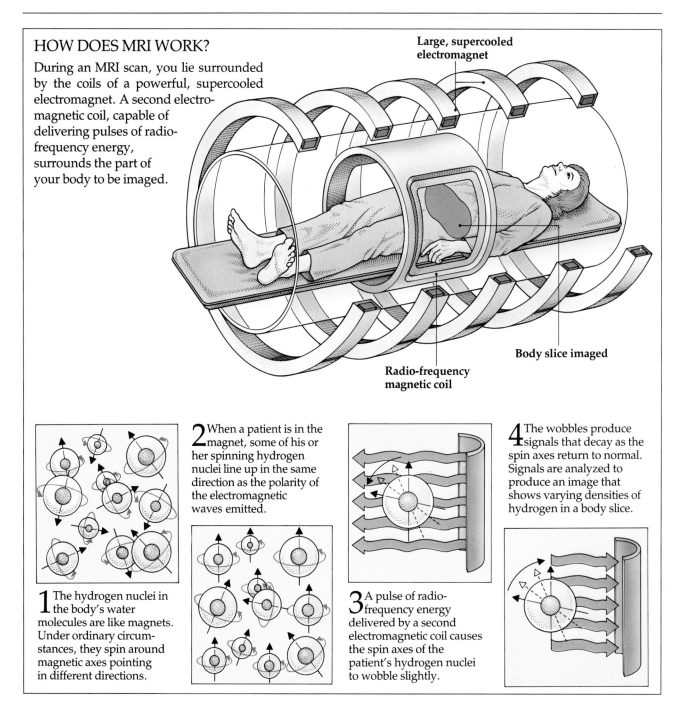

Large, supercooled electromagnet

Body slice imaged

Radio-frequency magnetic coil

1 The hydrogen nuclei in the body's water molecules are like magnets. Under ordinary circumstances, they spin around magnetic axes pointing in different directions.

2 When a patient is in the magnet, some of his or her spinning hydrogen nuclei line up in the same direction as the polarity of the electromagnetic waves emitted.

3 A pulse of radio-frequency energy delivered by a second electromagnetic coil causes the spin axes of the patient's hydrogen nuclei to wobble slightly.

4 The wobbles produce signals that decay as the spin axes return to normal. Signals are analyzed to produce an image that shows varying densities of hydrogen in a body slice.

strength and location of the signals. Today's MRI scanners operate on the nuclei of hydrogen atoms. Because hydrogen is present in water and in a variety of other substances that make up a large proportion of the body, almost the entire structure of the body can be imaged. Tissues that contain a great deal of hydrogen, such as fat, produce a bright image; those that contain less hydrogen, such as bone, appear darker.

DIAGNOSTIC USES

Unlike some other imaging techniques, MRI provides clear images of parts of the body surrounded by dense bone, making it particularly valuable for studying the brain and spinal cord. MRI can focus on details in the brain and spinal cord so delicate that it can even show the "scarring" of the covering of nerve fibers that

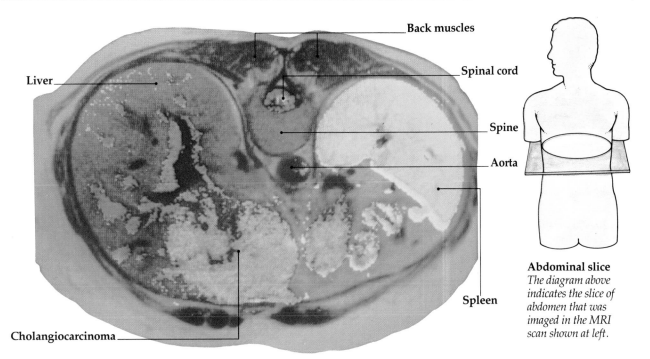

Back muscles

Spinal cord

Liver

Spine

Aorta

Spleen

Cholangiocarcinoma

Abdominal slice
The diagram above indicates the slice of abdomen that was imaged in the MRI scan shown at left.

MRI scan of abdomen
This color-enhanced scan shows a slice through the abdomen (shown as if you were looking from the top of the body downward). The patient was found to be suffering from a large cholangiocarcinoma (type of liver cancer), which is clearly visible as the orange mass in the scan. Also visible are the spine, spinal cord, spleen, aorta, and muscles of the back.

occurs in multiple sclerosis. It detects brain tumors more accurately than any other scanning method and indicates the extent to which they have invaded the brain. For example, if a person had a tumor in the lower back part of the skull (where the skull bones are likely to obscure a tumor), even a CT scan might fail to reveal it. However, because MRI is unaffected by overlying bone, the tumor can be seen. MRI is also useful for examining joints and soft tissues, particularly those in the knee.

MRI can also provide precise images of the heart and major blood vessels and gives a detailed picture of blood flow. It reveals blood in arteries and veins and contrasts it well with surrounding tissue. It can detect changes in the thickness of the heart muscle following a heart attack and can image congenital heart disease abnormalities. MRI also demonstrates disease-related changes that occur in body tissues. The technique can often distinguish normal brain tissue from areas of the brain that have been partially deprived of their blood supply, which occurs in a person who has had a stroke.

The images produced by MRI are similar to those produced by CT scanning (see page 48), but MRI generally provides a much greater contrast between normal and abnormal tissue. Also, MRI provides flexibility by virtue of its ability to scan the patient in any plane (e.g., vertically or crosswise).

How is it done?

MRI is usually an outpatient procedure. If you undergo MRI, you must lie very still during the examination. Children sometimes are given a general anesthetic. The scanner itself is an enormous hollow electromagnet. Although it appears imposingly large, part of its bulk is taken up by apparatus designed to cool the coils of the magnet during operation.

There is nothing to be apprehensive about if your doctor recommends MRI. You will not feel pain and the examination should be over in 45 to 60 minutes or less. All you will hear is the clicking sound of the machinery. About 10 percent of patients suffer feelings of claustrophobia during a scan. If you feel anxious about the procedure, talk to your doctor about it beforehand.

Because your body will be placed in a strong magnetic field, it is extremely important that you not carry any metallic

CASE HISTORY
A WORRISOME HEADACHE

KATIE'S MOTHER was getting increasingly concerned about her daughter's constant complaint of a headache. Katie had always been a healthy child, aside from the usual childhood illnesses, and her headache was a totally unexpected problem. At first, Katie's mother attributed the headache to changing schools. However, when Katie told her that her vision was "like seeing twice," Katie's mother became alarmed and made an appointment with her doctor that day.

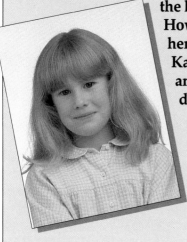

PERSONAL DETAILS
Name Katie Carter
Age 6
Occupation Schoolgirl
Family Both parents are in good health.

MEDICAL BACKGROUND
Other than the usual childhood illnesses, such as chickenpox, measles, and an occasional cold, Katie has always been healthy.

THE CONSULTATION
Katie's doctor notices that Katie looks pale and drawn. She also appears disoriented. Soon after entering the doctor's office, Katie runs to the sink and vomits, but seems to recover quickly and apologizes.

The doctor's questions establish that Katie has had a severe headache for the past 3 weeks. Katie tells the doctor that when she looks to her left her vision is normal, but when she looks to her right she sees "everything twice."

The doctor asks her to keep her head still and follow his finger with her eyes. When she looks to the left, her eyes move normally. However, when she looks to the right, her right eye does not move beyond the midline of her vision. The doctor concludes that the muscle that moves Katie's right eye outward is paralyzed, which accounts for the double vision. The doctor then puts some drops in Katie's eyes to enlarge her pupils. After half an hour, he examines the inside of her eyes with an ophthalmoscope. The doctor is concerned that the nerve heads of both optic nerves are noticeably swollen, bulging forward into the interior of Katie's eyes. He tells Katie's mother that her symptoms of headache and vomiting, and his own observations, indicate increased pressure inside Katie's skull. The doctor recommends going to the hospital immediately for a variety of diagnostic studies, including an MRI scan.

THE INVESTIGATION
Katie is old enough to be relieved that something is being done about her headache so she cooperates during the scan. She is a little frightened, though, when she is moved into the circular opening in the huge machine and is worried by the noise it makes. After Katie's mother reassures her that she won't feel any pain, Katie lies very still and excellent scans are obtained that reveal the problem immediately.

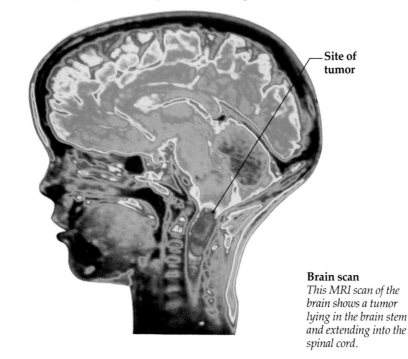

Site of tumor

Brain scan
This MRI scan of the brain shows a tumor lying in the brain stem and extending into the spinal cord.

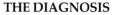

THE DIAGNOSIS

Katie has a brain stem TUMOR in the lower part of her skull that extends into her spinal cord. The tumor is near the surface of her brain stem, and the specialists are happy to see that it seems to be separate from the normal brain stem substance. The tumor is interfering with the circulation of the cerebrospinal fluid and elevating its pressure, which is causing her optic nerve heads to swell. The increased pressure inside her skull also accounts for her symptoms of double vision.

Katie's scan shows that the tumor is almost certainly malignant. However, the tumor is well localized, which means there is at least a 70 percent chance of a complete cure if surgery is performed early.

THE TREATMENT

Katie is operated on the next day. The operation takes 5 hours, during which the surgeon's primary goal is to remove as little of Katie's normal brain tissue as possible while removing the tumor completely. The surgery is made easier because the tumor has compressed the brain as opposed to invading the substance of the brain itself.

Katie makes a steady recovery and is able to get out of bed in 3 days, though she feels a little shaky at first and has a tendency to lurch to one side when she walks.

THE OUTCOME

Two weeks after the operation, Katie has apparently made a complete recovery. She has not had a headache or been vomiting, her eye movements are normal, and she is not seeing double anymore.

Katie is lucky. After 3 years, there is no recurrence of any of her previous symptoms. All follow-up MRI scans are normal.

Spinal cord tumor
The image at right shows a color-enhanced MRI scan of the upper chest, head, and neck of a young girl who was suffering from paralysis in her legs. It reveals clearly a tumor (in red) in the spinal cord. The information obtained from the scan allowed surgeons to remove the tumor, and the girl was able to walk again.

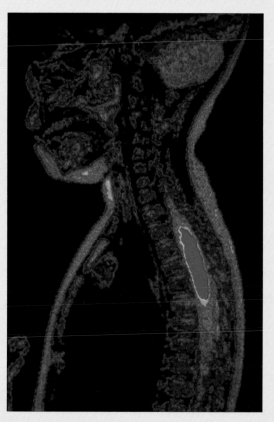

articles or wear any metal jewelry. In addition, tell your doctor if you have any metal implants such as an artificial hip joint, metal plates or screws in your bones, surgical clips, or any electrical device such as a pacemaker or hearing aid, which could be affected by the magnet.

INTERPRETATION

Doctors seeing an MRI scan for the first time could be forgiven for thinking that they are looking at photographs of cross-sectional body specimens from an anatomical museum, so detailed are the representations. Subtle abnormalities are revealed, and disorders of body function that do not cause structural alteration can be detected in many cases. The findings of an MRI scan – especially in the brain – are generally highly accurate.

Are there any risks?

MRI is not believed to be associated with any risks or side effects. It does not use ionizing radiation and can therefore be performed repeatedly without producing any known adverse effects.

NEW TYPES OF MRI

Until now, most MRI scanners have operated on the basis of detecting hydrogen atoms – a constituent of water that occurs in varying concentrations throughout the body tissues. However, scanners are also being developed, or are in use, that operate by detecting the atoms of other elements in the body. Phosphorus atoms, for example, are the usual basis for MRI scans of the muscle. These scans can be used to assess the function of muscle in the heart and elsewhere in the body.

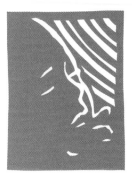

ULTRASOUND SCANNING

SINCE THE 1970S, many X-ray techniques have been superseded by newer procedures that are safer, simpler to perform, and more comfortable for the patient. Ultrasound scanning, which works by passing high-frequency sound waves through the body, today is the first choice for diagnostic imaging of the gallbladder, female genital tract, parts of the heart, and fetus. Doctors also use ultrasound scanning to image many other parts of the body.

An abdominal ultrasound scan
Ultrasound scanning is used to image many organs. It is a safe and effective imaging tool. Below, a patient is shown having an abdominal ultrasound scan.

The principle of ultrasound scanning is similar to that of marine sonar, in which sound waves are bounced off objects deep in the ocean. Also called sonography, ultrasound scanning is a technology that was derived from the naval sonar that was used to detect submarines during World War II.

HOW IT WORKS

Ultrasound waves are emitted by a device called a transducer, which is positioned on the skin over the part of the body to be viewed. The transducer contains a piezoelectric crystal, which converts an electrical current into high-frequency sound waves that can be focused into a narrow beam (the sound waves are too high pitched to be heard by the human ear).

If the transducer is moved back and forth, this beam passes through a "slice" of the body. Some of the waves are reflected by tissue boundaries, so a series of echoes is returned. The transducer also acts as a receiver, converting these echoes into electrical signals that are processed and displayed on a screen to give a two-dimensional image of the scanned body slice.

Modern ultrasound scanners display a continuously updated image. This means they are able to show movements within the body slice being scanned, such as fetal movements in the uterus.

IMAGING A KIDNEY CYST

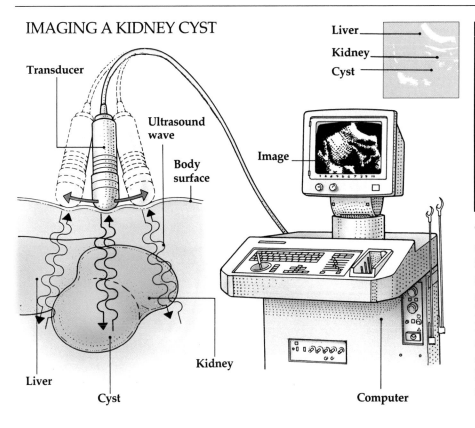

Transducer

Ultrasound wave

Body surface

Image

Liver

Cyst

Kidney

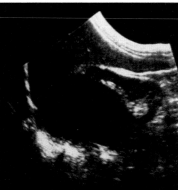

Liver

Kidney

Cyst

Computer

The diagram at left shows the organs that have been imaged in the ultrasound scan shown above. A large cyst is visible as a dark area in the right kidney. Part of the liver is also visible. In ultrasound scans, fluid-filled organs or cysts appear dark (no echoes), while organ or tissue boundaries appear bright (many echoes).

DIAGNOSTIC USES

Ultrasound waves pass readily through fluids and soft tissues, making them particularly useful for examining fluid-filled organs, such as the gallbladder and the pregnant uterus, and soft organs, such as the liver. Ultrasound waves do not, however, pass through bone or gas, so they are of limited use for examining parts of the body that are surrounded by bone, such as the brain, or that contain gas, such as the lungs or intestines.

One of the most common uses of ultrasound is to view the uterus and fetus in pregnancy (see SCREENING THE UNBORN BABY on page 122). It also has many nonobstetric uses. Ultrasound is widely used in heart imaging (see ECHOCARDIOGRAPHY on page 64). It is also valuable in the investigation of various conditions affecting the abdominal organs. Ultrasound may aid in or confirm a diagnosis of kidney cysts or tumors or hydronephrosis (a condition in which the collecting ducts of the kidneys are enlarged); diseases of the pancreas, such as tumors and pseudocysts; gallstones in, or inflammation of, the gallbladder; enlargement of the spleen or rupture of the spleen after major injury; and liver disorders such as liver enlargement, tumors, jaundice, cirrhosis, cysts, abscesses, and bile duct abnormalities. Other organs that may be scanned by ultrasound for diagnostic purposes, primarily to evaluate cysts, solid tumors, or foreign bodies, include the thyroid gland, breasts, bladder, testes, ovaries, spleen, and eyes.

Ultrasound can be used to scan the brain of a newborn, via the soft spot in the skull known as the fontanelle, to investigate hydrocephalus (water on the brain), and to diagnose a brain tumor or brain hemorrhage. The technique can also be used to measure blood flow through arteries in most parts of the body (see DOPPLER SCANNING on page 65). Ultrasound is especially effective in displaying movement within the body and

Twins revealed by ultrasound
Ultrasound scanning may be performed during pregnancy to check on the health of the fetus. The color-enhanced scan at right clearly shows twins in the uterus.

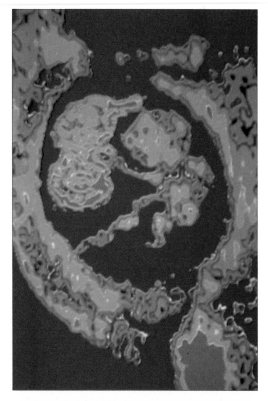

Scan showing an ovarian cyst
This ultrasound scan of a woman's abdomen reveals a large, fluid-filled cyst in one of her ovaries. The cyst appears as a large, dark area. Also visible in the scan are her bladder and, underneath the bladder, her uterus. The cyst was later successfully removed.

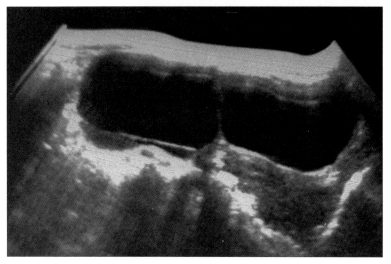

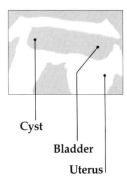

Cyst

Bladder

Uterus

in determining depth, which helps the doctor guide a needle accurately to a specific spot to withdraw a fluid sample or to guide the insertion of a catheter.

How is it done?

Before having an ultrasound scan, clothing over the area to be scanned is removed and jelly is smeared over the skin to achieve good contact as the transducer is passed back and forth over the skin. A scan takes between 15 and 30 minutes.

For many types of scans, you lie down on an examination table near the ultrasound machine; the room is darkened so that images on the screen can be seen more clearly. The machine produces vibrations well above the level we can hear or feel so, apart from the slight pressure of the transducer head on your skin, you will feel nothing.

There are many different kinds of ultrasound machines. For certain examinations you may be asked to sit comfortably in a chair while the ultrasound test is being done. Ultrasound examination of the eye may sound alarming, but, if your doctor recommends this procedure, there is no reason for concern. For ocular ultrasound, the transducer used is very small and is pressed gently against your closed eyelid.

For a liver or gallbladder scan, you are asked to fast for 12 hours beforehand to minimize the amount of gas in the intestine, which interferes with ultrasound transmission. For examination of the fetus or pelvic area, a full bladder is necessary. Consequently, you will be asked to drink three or four glasses of water 20 to 30 minutes before the test.

INTERPRETATION

To interpret ultrasound pictures meaningfully, the doctor or ultrasound technician must bear in mind that the images he or she is viewing are representations of reflections from surfaces that are exactly perpendicular to the ultrasound beam. Only a single plane is in view at any time. Surfaces at an angle to this plane may appear as wavy lines because the plane cuts through them. If the doctor chooses, he or she can "freeze" image slices on the screen for closer examination, much like pressing the pause button on a video recording. The images can also be reproduced as photographs.

To those of us not used to seeing images of cross-sectional anatomy, ultrasound pictures may appear confusing –

CASE HISTORY
SEVERE ABDOMINAL PAIN

CYNTHIA HAS BEEN **troubled by periods of severe pain in her upper abdomen for the past 48 hours. The pain first appeared abruptly, lasted for about 10 minutes, and stopped as suddenly as it started, leaving her feeling nauseated, alarmed, and anxious. On the second occasion, she also vomited and had a pain under her right shoulder blade.**

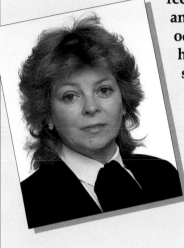

PERSONAL DETAILS
Name Cynthia Richardson
Age 44
Occupation Advertising executive
Family Cynthia's father died of stomach cancer.

MEDICAL BACKGROUND
Cynthia is an active, energetic woman, popular with her colleagues and highly successful at her work. She has always had a weight problem. However, despite repeated dieting, she has remained well above her ideal weight.

THE CONSULTATION
Cynthia tells the doctor that, for several months, she has had discomfort in her upper abdomen. She has also noticed that certain kinds of food tend to give her indigestion. Cynthia's father died of stomach cancer. She is convinced that cancer is the cause of her recent, severe, abdominal pains, and that the cancer has already spread to the back of her chest.

During a conversation with her doctor, Cynthia remembers that there were times when her bowel movements looked unusually pale, but she says she did not think it was important. The doctor checks her temperature and finds it normal. He then applies pressure with his hands at different spots on her abdomen and discovers an area of tenderness on her right side.

THE DOCTOR'S IMPRESSION
Cynthia's symptoms, in addition to her age, gender, and weight, point to a problem with her gallbladder. The doctor refers her to the local hospital for an ultrasound scan. She is instructed to fast for 12 hours before the scan is performed.

FURTHER INVESTIGATION
The ultrasound examination lasts for about 20 minutes. During the course of the scan, Cynthia is periodically asked to hold her breath; she watches the technician make some marks on her abdomen with a felt-tipped pen to pinpoint areas of interest.

THE DIAGNOSIS
The ultrasound scan reveals that Cynthia's gallbladder contains a large GALLSTONE. The pain Cynthia has been experiencing was due to the passage of smaller stones through the bile duct that links the liver and gallbladder to the intestine.

The area of tenderness over her abdomen corresponds with the location of the gallbladder. Her indigestion after eating high-fat meals may be related to dysfunction of the gallbladder. Her pain may be due in part to contractions of the gallbladder triggered by fat or stomach acid entering the intestine.

THE TREATMENT
Obstruction of the duct that leads from the gallbladder can be dangerous and can lead to inflammation of the wall of the gallbladder, to a large collection of pus in the gallbladder, or to gangrene in part of the wall of the gallbladder. Cynthia's doctor advises her to have her gallbladder removed. At the same time, the surgeon will explore her common bile duct for gallstones and drain the duct itself. After the operation, she experiences no more symptoms.

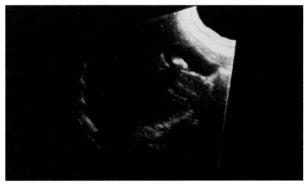

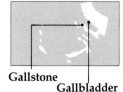

Gallstone
Gallbladder
Confirmation
An ultrasound scan of Cynthia's abdomen confirms the presence of a gallstone in her gallbladder.

somewhat like blurred photographs. However, an experienced doctor can derive a great deal of information from an ultrasound picture.

When the procedure is over, the radiologist will discuss the results of your scan with your doctor. In general, the findings of a scan are highly accurate.

Are there any risks?

The advantage of ultrasound imaging is its high level of safety, which means it can be used repeatedly without causing harm. Ultrasound scanning has been in use for more than a quarter of a century without producing evidence of risk.

ECHOCARDIOGRAPHY

Echocardiography uses ultrasound to allow the doctor to visualize the internal structure of the heart and its movements. The transducer is placed on the surface of the chest and the beam is directed to various parts of the heart. By moving the transducer systematically over the heart area, a detailed picture is gradually constructed.

Echocardiography is useful in showing abnormalities of the heart valves, such as defects in the mitral or aortic valves, which are particularly prone to disease. If your doctor finds a heart murmur that he or she suspects is caused by a mitral valve disorder, echocardiography often reveals that the murmur is due to a slight and often harmless ballooning of one or more of the leaflets of this valve. Called mitral valve leaflet prolapse, it can sometimes be significant. However, more often than not, this is not the case. An ultrasound scan can help make the distinction.

Echocardiography can also show all types of congenital (present from birth) heart disease and can readily detect defects of heart wall motion, bulging of the heart wall (aneurysm), and rare tumors, called myxomas, that can form inside the heart (usually in an atrium).

HOW ECHOCARDIOGRAPHY WORKS

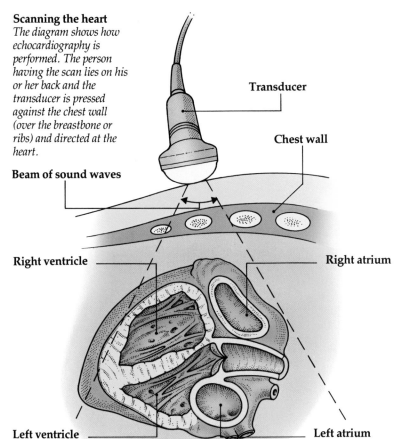

Scanning the heart
The diagram shows how echocardiography is performed. The person having the scan lies on his or her back and the transducer is pressed against the chest wall (over the breastbone or ribs) and directed at the heart.

Transducer

Chest wall

Beam of sound waves

Right ventricle

Right atrium

Left ventricle

Left atrium

Echocardiogram
The echoes from the structures in the heart are analyzed to construct an image such as that shown at right. All four of the heart chambers (two atria and two ventricles) are clearly visible here. This type of image is useful for diagnosing defects in the heart chambers and valves.

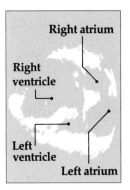

Right atrium

Right ventricle

Left ventricle

Left atrium

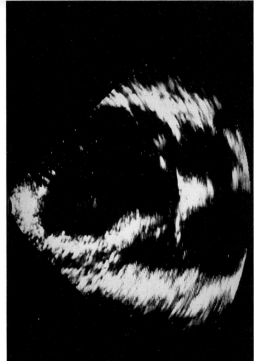

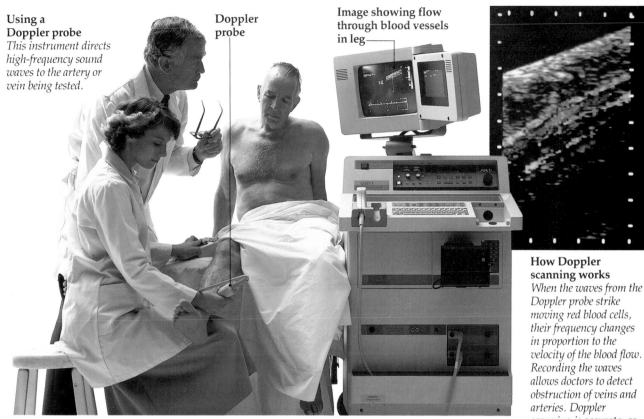

Using a Doppler probe
This instrument directs high-frequency sound waves to the artery or vein being tested.

Doppler probe

Image showing flow through blood vessels in leg

How Doppler scanning works
When the waves from the Doppler probe strike moving red blood cells, their frequency changes in proportion to the velocity of the blood flow. Recording the waves allows doctors to detect obstruction of veins and arteries. Doppler scanning is accurate, as well as being safer, quicker, and less costly than invasive tests.

The scan at top right, of the blood flow through part of a patient's leg, shows a typical image produced by Doppler scanning. Fast-flowing arterial blood is color-coded in red and slower-flowing venous blood is blue.

DOPPLER SCANNING

Doppler scanning is a type of ultrasound scanning used to measure blood flow through the blood vessels. It is accurate and especially useful in investigating serious or potentially serious problems caused by inadequate blood supply to the legs or arms as a result of blood vessel disease. Doppler scanning can detect a substantial, endangering reduction in blood flow in 95 percent of cases.

How does it work?
The pitch of a note depends on its sound frequency. If the source of the sound is moving toward you or away from you, the frequency received changes, becoming higher with an approaching source and lower if the source is moving away. This principle, called the Doppler effect, explains why the pitch of a police siren or train seems to rise as the vehicle approaches and to drop when the vehicle has passed.

The same principle applies if there is movement of the surface from which sound waves are being reflected. This allows the Doppler effect to be used, in conjunction with ultrasound, to investigate the movement of columns of blood in blood vessels. It can also show turbulence in narrowed arteries, in opening and closing heart valves, and in movements of the heart muscle.

How is it done?
You will be asked to lie down, move your arms or legs, and breathe deeply as measurements are taken, to vary the flow of blood during the examination. The blood flow is measured with a Doppler probe, a hand-held transducer that directs high-frequency sound waves to the artery or vein being tested. In recent years, conventional ultrasound imaging and Doppler technology have been combined. Duplex Doppler ultrasound provides doctors with images that show the anatomy and structure of organs as well as the flow of blood through the vessels.

CHAPTER FOUR

LIGHT AND ELECTRICAL TESTS

INTRODUCTION

ENDOSCOPY

EYE EXAMINATIONS

ELECTRICAL TESTS

HEARING TESTS

N OT ALL DIAGNOSTIC tests rely on sophisticated scanners or complex chemical and microanalytical techniques. Some procedures are more fundamental. Foremost among these simpler tests are direct observation using light and a variety of examinations using electricity. The first part of this chapter describes the light-conducting viewing instruments known as endoscopes. Developed in the early part of this century (after pioneering efforts using professional sword swallowers), the original endoscopes were simple, rigid, open tubes. These early versions have been largely replaced by far more sophisticated, flexible endoscopes that can be maneuvered around corners and past obstructions inside the body. Fiberoptic endoscopes are a classic example of modern technological wizardry. These plastic tubes are usually little thicker than a pencil and are tightly packed with channels that conduct air, water, biopsy attachments, control wires, and groups of optical fibers. Most doctors who use endoscopes would confirm that the view through the instrument is not always clear. In addition, using an endoscope requires manual dexterity. However, these devices allow direct observation of disease processes in natural color – a real

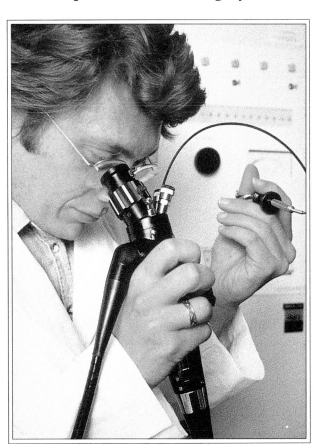

advantage over X-ray imaging techniques. Video attachments enable the doctor to see internal structures on a screen and to keep a permanent record of the examination. Your brain, nerves, sense organs, and muscles function by means of the most complex electrochemical cabling, transmission, processing, and signaling system imaginable. Your heart has a self-contained, and highly efficient, electrical system of its own. As explained in the section of this chapter on electrical tests, many disorders of these organs can now be investigated by looking for anomalies in their electrical activity or responsiveness. Many heart disorders, for example, leave a characteristic "fingerprint" in a graphic tracing of the heart's electrical activity (an electrocardiogram). The printouts from electrocardiography and other electrical tests may appear as no more than a confusing series of wavy lines on graph paper. However, to the trained diagnostician, the printouts provide vital clues to the diagnosis of such diverse disorders as holes in the heart, multiple sclerosis, and epilepsy. Also included in this chapter are sections on the specialized optical, microscopic, fiberoptic, and electronic equipment now used by doctors in the process of diagnosing sight and hearing disorders.

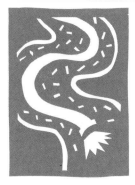

ENDOSCOPY

Unlike other diagnostic tools, endoscopes allow doctors to see, with their own eyes, what is taking place inside your body. Endoscopy enables a doctor to confirm a diagnosis, monitor a condition, and in some cases even treat a problem, all without the need to perform a more invasive surgical procedure.

How fiberoptic endoscopes work
Light travels down the illuminating fiberoptic bundles in straight lines, "bouncing" from one side of each fiber to the other. The viewing fibers are strictly organized so that, when light reflects back up the endoscope from the area being examined, a coherent image is formed at the eyepiece of the instrument.

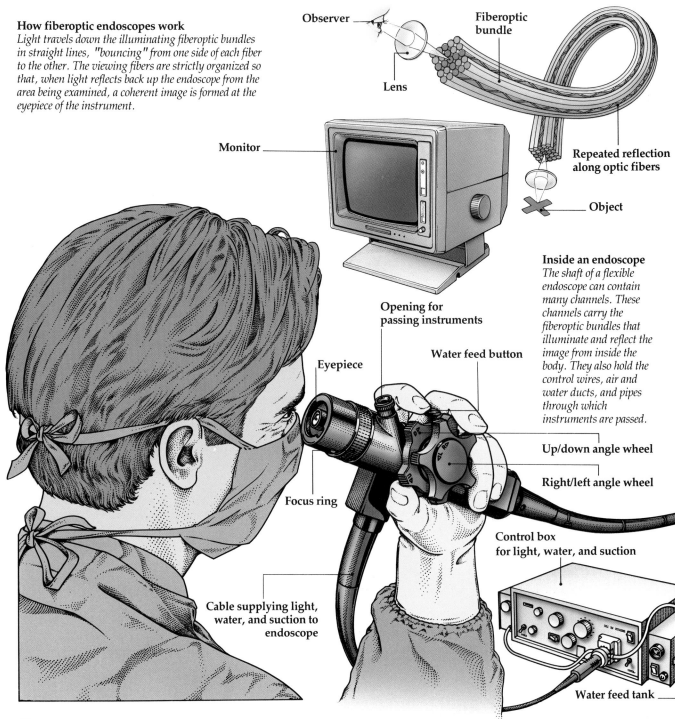

Observer

Fiberoptic bundle

Lens

Repeated reflection along optic fibers

Monitor

Object

Inside an endoscope
The shaft of a flexible endoscope can contain many channels. These channels carry the fiberoptic bundles that illuminate and reflect the image from inside the body. They also hold the control wires, air and water ducts, and pipes through which instruments are passed.

Opening for passing instruments

Water feed button

Eyepiece

Up/down angle wheel

Right/left angle wheel

Focus ring

Control box for light, water, and suction

Cable supplying light, water, and suction to endoscope

Water feed tank

The endoscope is an optical instrument that is introduced into your body to visually examine the structures inside. Although several types of rigid metal endoscopes are still in use, most of today's endoscopes are fiberoptic, consisting of a pencil-thin plastic tube that contains flexible bundles of plastic or glass fibers. A powerful light is shined down one bundle of fibers to illuminate the area of the body being tested. The image is reflected back up the tube along another bundle of fibers and magnified by a lens in the eyepiece. A flexible endoscope can be maneuvered around corners and into position, and instruments can be passed down the endoscope to remove polyps (growths) or to take samples of any tissue that appears abnormal. Newer endoscopes employ miniature television cameras, allowing the doctor to view internal structures on a large monitor and record the images.

ENDOSCOPIC ATTACHMENTS

A variety of specialized tools can be passed through an endoscope's instrument channel for taking samples of tissue or cells and for such minor operations as polyp removal.

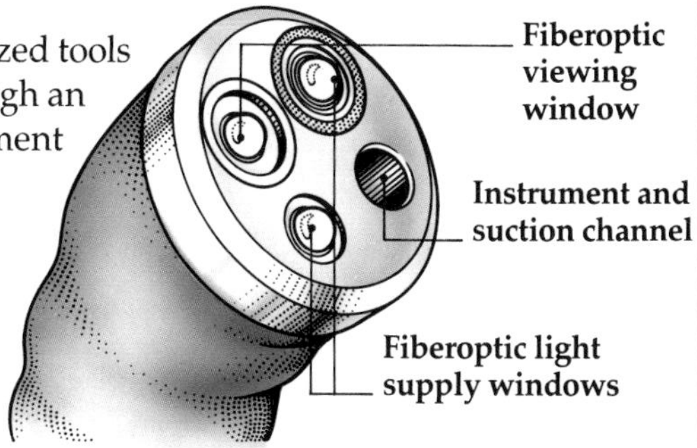

Fiberoptic viewing window

Instrument and suction channel

Fiberoptic light supply windows

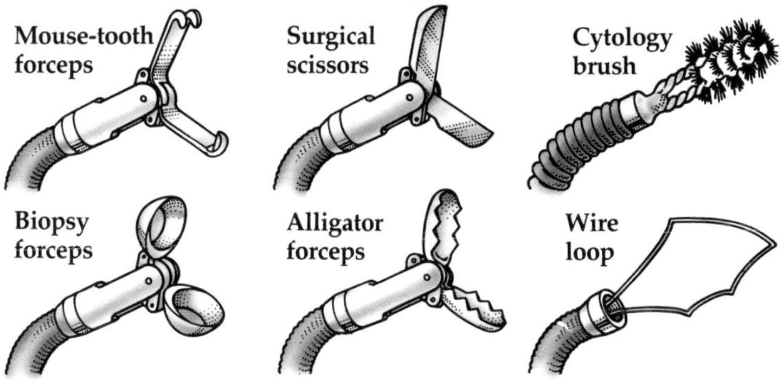

Mouse-tooth forceps

Surgical scissors

Cytology brush

Biopsy forceps

Alligator forceps

Wire loop

WHAT THE DOCTOR SEES

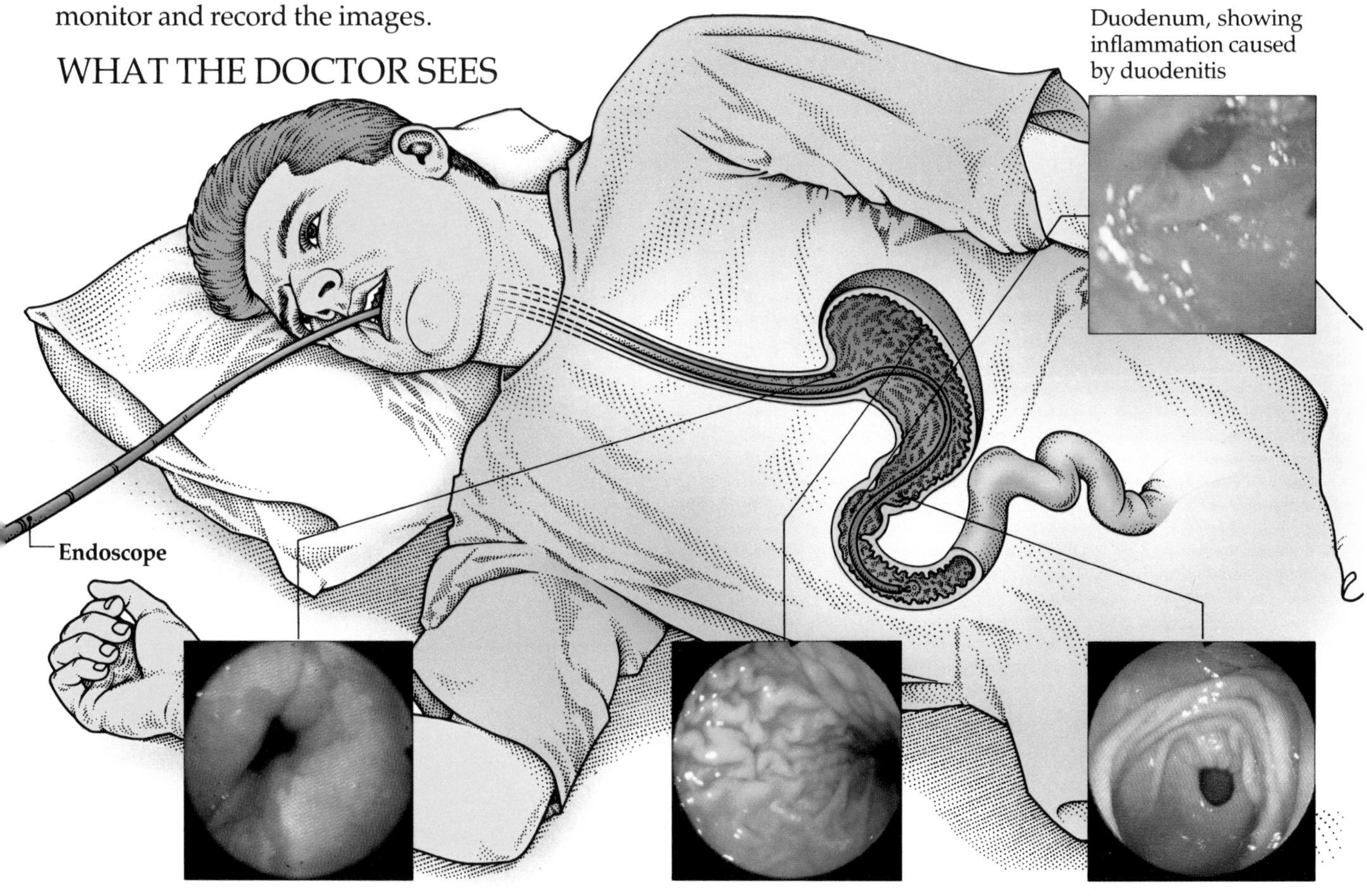

Endoscope

Duodenum, showing inflammation caused by duodenitis

Junction of the esophagus and stomach

Folds in the lining of the stomach

Junction of the stomach and duodenum

The gastrointestinal tract is by far the most common subject of endoscopic examination. If your esophagus, stomach, or duodenum (first part of the small intestine) is to be examined, the instrument is inserted through your mouth. The colon (main part of the large intestine), rectum, and anal canal are viewed with longer endoscopes, which the doctor inserts through your anus.

ESOPHAGOSCOPY AND GASTRODUODENOSCOPY

These examinations are usually performed in the special procedures room in the hospital; they take about half an hour. Your doctor may be trying to locate the cause of swallowing difficulty, heartburn, ulcerlike pain, or persistent indigestion that has been unresponsive to treatment. If you have vomited blood, the endoscopy may be able to pinpoint the source of the internal bleeding.

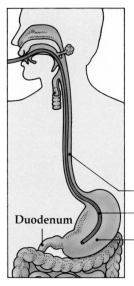

Examining the upper digestive tract
During esophagoscopy and gastroduodenoscopy, the doctor passes an endoscope down the back of your throat into your esophagus. In gastroduodenoscopy, the endoscope is passed farther down into the stomach and duodenum.

— **Esophagus**

— **Endoscope**

Duodenum

— **Stomach**

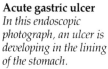

Acute gastric ulcer
In this endoscopic photograph, an ulcer is developing in the lining of the stomach.

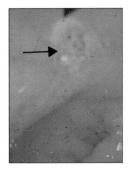

PREPARING FOR AN ENDOSCOPIC EXAMINATION

A gastrointestinal endoscopy performed at the hospital or your doctor's office may require the following:

Transportation home
Arrange for someone to drive you home; you will probably feel drowsy for several hours after the examination.

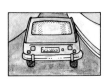

Clearing the tract
♦ The night before a colonoscopy you may take a strong laxative. Before the examination an enema may also be given or a liquid laxative alone may be used to cleanse the colon.
♦ Before a sigmoidoscopy or a proctoscopy you may be required to empty your rectum with the assistance of a suppository or an enema.

Food and fluids
What you eat and drink before an endoscopy depends on the type of examination to be performed.
♦ No food or fluids are allowed for 6 hours before an esophagoscopy or a gastroduodenoscopy.
♦ Before a colonoscopy or a sigmoidoscopy diets vary.

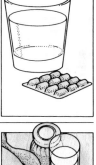

Consent
It is customary for a doctor or nurse to explain the endoscopic procedure to you, after which you sign a consent form.

Dress
You will be asked to remove your clothes, along with any jewelry and dentures, and put on a hospital gown.

Body position
If the endoscope is to be introduced by mouth, you may lie on your left side. For a bowel examination it is common to lie on your left side with your knees drawn up toward you. The endoscope is introduced through your anus.

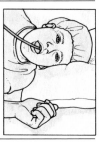

Esophagoscopy helps identify inflammation caused by esophagitis, ulceration, tumor, obstruction due to a stricture (abnormal narrowing of a passage) or foreign body, dilated veins, hiatal hernia (in which the stomach bulges up through the diaphragm into the chest), or abnormal muscle contractions. Gastroduodenoscopy can help identify the inflammation of gastritis and duodenitis, gastric or duodenal ulcers, scarring at the gastric outlet, benign tumors, malignant tumors (such as stomach cancer), or a foreign body that has been swallowed.

Medication is usually given about an hour before the procedure to help you relax and to reduce the secretions in your mouth and stomach. If a flexible endoscope is used, you will be given an intravenous injection of a sedative to make you feel sleepy, but it is common to remain partially conscious throughout the procedure. A local anesthetic will also be given, either as a gargle or sprayed onto the back of your throat, to reduce any discomfort or gagging associated with the procedure.

How are the tests done?

The doctor places a finger in your mouth to guide the tip of the endoscope; you will be asked to swallow as the endoscope is passed down the back of your throat. A mouth guard is usually inserted between your teeth to prevent you from biting the endoscope. During gastroduodenoscopy you may be aware that the endoscope is being moved around in your stomach. You may also have a feeling of fullness when air is introduced into the digestive tract to separate the walls of the stomach.

After the examination you may feel a little light-headed as the intravenous sedation continues to wear off, and your throat will probably be a little sore. You will be asked not to eat or drink anything for several hours until your gag reflex returns, to make sure you don't choke or inhale liquids or solid food.

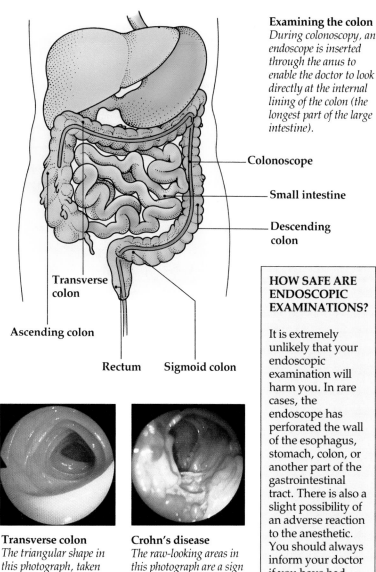

Examining the colon
During colonoscopy, an endoscope is inserted through the anus to enable the doctor to look directly at the internal lining of the colon (the longest part of the large intestine).

Colonoscope

Small intestine

Descending colon

Transverse colon

Ascending colon

Rectum   Sigmoid colon

Transverse colon
The triangular shape in this photograph, taken through a colonoscope, is typical of how the doctor views the transverse colon.

Crohn's disease
The raw-looking areas in this photograph are a sign of colonic Crohn's disease, a form of inflammatory bowel disease.

COLONOSCOPY

Colonoscopy, which takes about an hour, is performed in the special procedures room at the hospital. You will be given an intravenous injection of a sedative that will make you sleepy but you will remain conscious throughout the procedure. Colonoscopy helps identify the cause of lower abdominal pain, rectal or colonic bleeding, or persistent diarrhea. It can locate inflammation, ulceration, polyps, or tumors.

HOW SAFE ARE ENDOSCOPIC EXAMINATIONS?

It is extremely unlikely that your endoscopic examination will harm you. In rare cases, the endoscope has perforated the wall of the esophagus, stomach, colon, or another part of the gastrointestinal tract. There is also a slight possibility of an adverse reaction to the anesthetic. You should always inform your doctor if you have had such a reaction on a previous occasion.

If a biopsy is taken or a polyp removed, there may be some blood in your next bowel movement. You should tell your doctor if you have ever had problems with bleeding. Your doctor may want to perform another endoscopy several months to a year after removing a tumor or polyp to make sure there has been no recurrence.

TEST RESULTS

Before you leave the hospital or doctor's office, your doctor usually talks to you about the preliminary findings of the endoscopic examination (unless you are still drowsy). Samples taken from the area under investigation will be sent to a laboratory; the results of the laboratory analysis are usually not known for several days.

Examining the lower bowel
Sigmoidoscopy is performed to view the internal lining of the sigmoid colon and rectum. If a flexible sigmoidoscope is used, part of the descending colon can sometimes be viewed as well. Proctoscopy allows the doctor to view the internal lining of the anal canal and lower rectum.

How is the test done?

First, the doctor inserts a gloved, lubricated finger to ensure that there is no obstruction to the passage of the colonoscope. The colonoscope is then lubricated and gently inserted through the anus. It may feel cold and give you the sensation that you are going to move your bowels. You will be asked to breathe deeply and slowly through your mouth to relax your abdominal muscles.

Your doctor may move you into different positions on the examination table and may press your abdomen to help guide the colonoscope up the intestine. The colonoscope is then withdrawn slowly so the doctor can examine each part of the intestine as it comes into view. Once the colonoscope is removed, you will need to rest lying down for a while. Though you will feel light-headed at first, you can eat and drink as soon as you are fully conscious.

SIGMOIDOSCOPY AND PROCTOSCOPY

Both these examinations can be performed in the doctor's office. Sigmoidoscopy takes up to 30 minutes; proctoscopy takes only a few minutes.

The reasons for these examinations are broadly the same as for colonoscopy, but they are used primarily for checking disorders lower down in the digestive tract. In addition, the proctoscope may reveal hemorrhoids or an anal fissure.

How are the tests done?

Because the procedures cause very little physical discomfort, sedation is recommended only if you are extremely anxious about the test. However, a local anesthetic cream or suppository may be used to deaden the anal canal if its lining is tender because of inflammation, or if there is a fissure in the canal.

The procedure for flexible sigmoidoscopy is identical to that for colonoscopy, although the endoscope used is about half as long and the examination usually takes less time to perform.

To perform proctoscopy, the doctor first uses a gloved, lubricated finger to ensure that there is no obstruction or tenderness. After gently inserting the lubricated proctoscope, the doctor may ask you to strain (as if you were moving your bowels) to make any hemorrhoids stand out more clearly. Each part of the intestinal lining is examined as the proctoscope is slowly withdrawn.

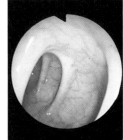

Sigmoid colon
Unlike the triangular transverse colon, the sigmoid colon has an oval configuration.

Ulcerative colitis
The pseudopolyps visible in this endoscopic photograph of the sigmoid colon are a healing stage of ulcerative colitis.

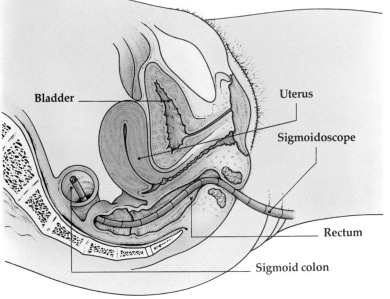

Bladder

Uterus

Sigmoidoscope

Rectum

Sigmoid colon

CASE HISTORY
PERSISTENT DIARRHEA

CRAIG HAD BEEN **suffering from diarrhea for the last 2 weeks. At first he had attributed it to a hamburger he had eaten at a ball game. When his condition did not improve, Craig thought the diarrhea might be due to all the stress he was under at work. He purchased an antidiarrheal medicine from a drugstore, but it was ineffective. When Craig saw blood in his stools he decided to call his doctor.**

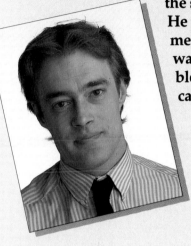

PERSONAL DETAILS
Name Craig Kelly
Age 28
Occupation Real estate broker
Family Father recently died of cancer of the bowel at age 62. Mother is healthy and active.

THE CONSULTATION
Craig tells the doctor that he has been moving his bowels 12 times a day and that there is blood in his stools. The stools have been loose, almost like water at times, and he has also been passing some mucus. The doctor examines Craig and finds no abdominal tenderness or masses in his abdomen. She asks Craig to lie on his side and performs an examination with her finger to see if there is any tenderness or swelling in Craig's lower rectum. Apart from a little blood on the glove, she finds nothing abnormal.

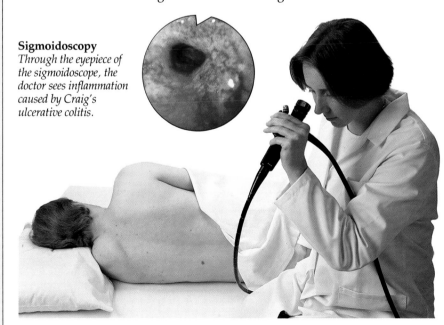

Sigmoidoscopy
Through the eyepiece of the sigmoidoscope, the doctor sees inflammation caused by Craig's ulcerative colitis.

FURTHER INVESTIGATION
The doctor decides to use a sigmoidoscope to look at the internal lining of Craig's colon. Through the eyepiece the doctor can see that the lining of the rectum and lower sigmoid colon is inflamed. A cotton swab passed through the sigmoidoscope and rubbed gently against the lining causes it to bleed. The doctor takes a biopsy from the inflamed lining and a swab from the stools to send to the laboratory for microscopic examination for parasites. The stool will also be cultured to see if an infection is causing the inflammation and diarrhea.

THE DIAGNOSIS
The biopsy report confirms that Craig is suffering from ULCERATIVE COLITIS, an uncommon condition of unknown cause that results in inflammation and ulceration of the lining of the colon and rectum. The condition causes increased mucus and fluid secretion and some bleeding into the bowel, which accounts for Craig's bloody diarrhea. The microbiology report, when it is returned from the laboratory, shows no sign of infection.

THE TREATMENT
Craig is prescribed two oral anti-inflammatory medications and is given a steroid retention enema to insert into his rectum each day. The enema will help reduce the inflammation in his colon.

THE OUTLOOK
After 3 weeks, the diarrhea had cleared up, another sigmoidoscopic examination showed healing, and Craig was able to stop using the steroid enema and start reducing his daily dose of one of the anti-inflammatory drugs. He will continue taking the other drug for 6 months.

PERFORMING A LAPAROSCOPY

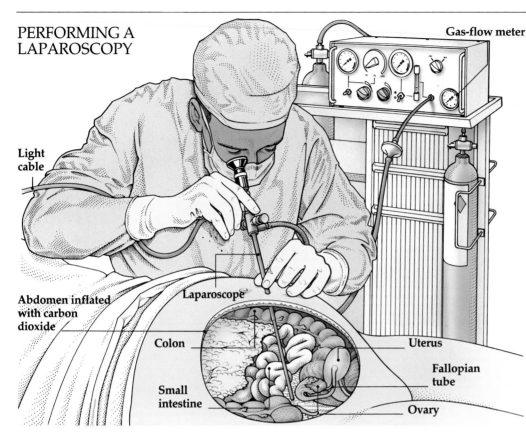

Gas-flow meter

Light cable

Abdomen inflated with carbon dioxide

Laparoscope

Colon

Small intestine

Uterus

Fallopian tube

Ovary

Examining the inside of the abdomen
In laparoscopy, an endoscope is inserted through the front of the abdomen to enable the doctor to view internal organs in the abdominal and pelvic cavities. Laparoscopy helps the doctor identify the cause of lower abdominal pain, pelvic pain, and pain during intercourse. It can confirm pelvic infection, tumors, cysts, fibroids, or an obstruction in the fallopian tubes.

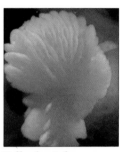

Fallopian tube
This photograph of the trumpet-shaped ending of the fallopian tube, the channel that conducts the egg from the ovary to the uterus, was taken during a laparoscopy.

The use of the endoscope as a diagnostic and surgical tool extends to many parts of the body, including the reproductive system, the respiratory tract, the urinary tract, and the inside of the joints.

LAPAROSCOPY

Laparoscopy, a technique for viewing the inside of the abdomen, is done on an outpatient basis; it takes about 30 minutes. A general anesthetic is given and you are positioned on your back with your knees bent and apart and your feet supported in stirrups.

How is the test done?
The doctor usually empties your bladder using a sterile catheter. After performing a pelvic examination, the doctor makes one or two small incisions in your navel and inserts a needle. Up to 3 liters of carbon dioxide gas are passed through the needle to distend the abdominal cavity. The laparoscope is then passed into the cavity to view the area being tested.

LARYNGOSCOPY

Laryngoscopy helps the doctor identify the cause of persistent hoarseness, loss of voice, and other voice disorders. It can reveal a polyp or tumor on the vocal cords or an obstruction due to a stricture or an inhaled foreign body. Laryngoscopy is also used to confirm the diagnosis of cancer of the larynx.

How is the test done?
You are given an injection of a sedative to help you relax and atropine to reduce the secretions in your throat and mouth. If you are not given a general anesthetic, a local anesthetic will be sprayed onto the back of your throat to reduce discomfort when the laryngoscope is inserted. You then lie flat or sit with your head held in position, and the laryngoscope is inserted into your throat.

After the examination, an ice pack may be applied to your throat to reduce the risk of swelling in the larynx. If a

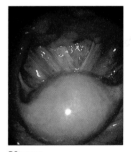

Uterus
The muscular organ in the foreground of this endoscopic photograph is the uterus; it is suspended in the pelvic cavity by ligaments and fibrous bands.

biopsy has been taken, you should try not to clear your throat or cough excessively because doing so could dislodge a blood clot and cause bleeding.

After a direct laryngoscopy you may experience a sore throat, hoarseness, or loss of voice, which usually goes away within the next day or two.

Direct laryngoscopy
A direct laryngoscopy (below) is performed when indirect laryngoscopy cannot provide a sufficiently detailed view. A rigid endoscope is inserted through your mouth and into the throat for close examination.

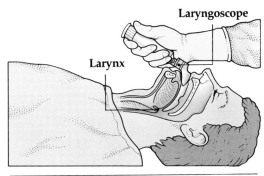

Indirect laryngoscopy
For indirect laryngoscopy (below), the doctor uses mirrors to look down your throat at your larynx and vocal cords.

Larynx
In this view of the vocal cords, no abnormality can be seen.

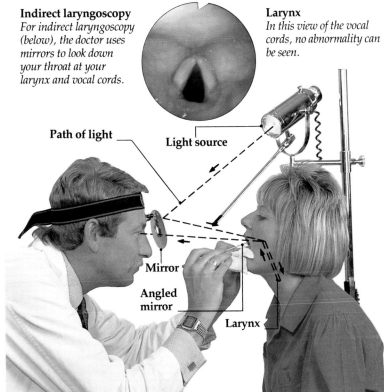

Path of light

Light source

Mirror

Angled mirror

Larynx

BRONCHOSCOPY

Bronchoscopy helps the doctor identify the cause of a persistent cough or coughing up blood. In addition to confirming the presence of an inhaled foreign body or a tumor and locating the source of any bleeding, bronchoscopy can also provide samples to be examined for signs of cancer or lung infection.

How is the test done?
You are first given an injection of a sedative in your arm; a topical anesthetic is applied to your throat. Under certain circumstances, a general anesthetic may be used. You then usually lie flat, but the procedure can be done while you sit upright. Before the bronchoscope is inserted, the tip is smeared with an anesthetic gel. The bronchoscope is then guided into each airway so your doctor can examine the lining of the bronchi. Samples may also be taken. In extremely rare cases, infection or a collapsed lung occurs after a bronchoscopy.

Examining the inside of the airway
There are two kinds of bronchoscopes – rigid (right) and flexible (below). During bronchoscopy, the endoscope is passed beyond the larynx into the trachea (windpipe) and into the bronchi (the large airways leading into the lungs).

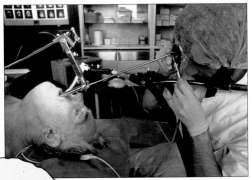

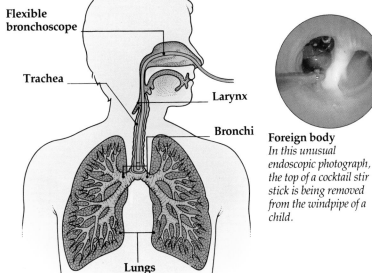

Flexible bronchoscope

Trachea

Larynx

Bronchi

Lungs

Foreign body
In this unusual endoscopic photograph, the top of a cocktail stir stick is being removed from the windpipe of a child.

CYSTOURETHROSCOPY

Cystourethroscopy helps the doctor identify the causes of blood in the urine and difficulty passing urine. It can confirm the presence of inflammation and tumors in the bladder and can pinpoint a stone or stricture in the urethra that is restricting the outflow of urine. Cystourethroscopy is also used in follow-up examinations for men who have undergone prostate gland surgery.

How is the test done?

You may be given a general anesthetic. If not, a local anesthetic gel is instilled into the urethra to reduce any discomfort when the cystourethroscope is inserted. You then lie on your back with your knees bent and apart and your feet supported in stirrups. You may have a slight burning sensation as the instrument is passed through the urethra. After the examination, you will be encouraged to drink plenty of fluids.

Examining the lower urinary tract
In cystourethroscopy, an endoscope is inserted into the urethra to enable the doctor to look directly at the internal lining of the urethra and bladder. A cystoscope is used to look inside the bladder; a urethroscope is used to examine the urethra and the neck of the bladder.

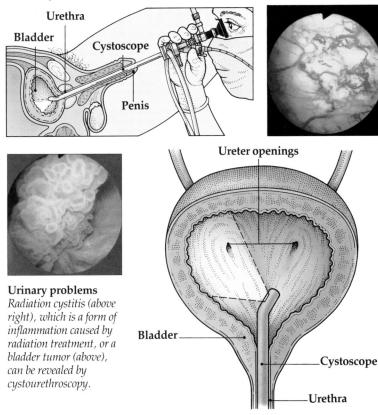

Urethra

Bladder

Cystoscope

Penis

Ureter openings

Bladder

Cystoscope

Urethra

Urinary problems
Radiation cystitis (above right), which is a form of inflammation caused by radiation treatment, or a bladder tumor (above), can be revealed by cystourethroscopy.

ASK YOUR DOCTOR
ENDOSCOPY

Q **Does an endoscope ever get caught or stuck when it is moving around inside the body?**

A No, the doctor using the endoscope is trained to maneuver it. If the endoscope can be passed around an obstruction or through a narrow opening, there is no reason it cannot be withdrawn along the same path.

Q **I had a barium X-ray last week, so why is my doctor saying that I must now have a gastroduodenoscopy?**

A It could be that your X-ray did not confirm a diagnosis. Gastroduodenoscopy shows the lining of the stomach and duodenum in better detail and it may pick up an abnormality that was invisible on the barium X-ray. Also, the endoscope will enable your doctor to take a sample of any questionable area.

Q **My husband has been referred for a mediastinoscopy. What does this examination involve?**

A In this procedure, an endoscope is inserted into the central compartment of the chest through an incision in the neck. It is done to find out more about enlarged lymph glands or a cyst or tumor seen on an X-ray.

Q **Will the gas that is put into my abdomen during laparoscopy cause any unpleasant symptoms?**

A Most of the gas is eliminated by the doctor gently pressing on your abdomen before removing the laparoscope sheath. While the small amount left may cause abdominal discomfort and some shoulder pain, the gas will be absorbed into your bloodstream over the next few days.

SEEING INSIDE A JOINT

In arthroscopy, an endoscope is inserted into a joint to look directly at the structures inside (right). The arthroscope is used most often to examine and treat the knee, shoulder, or ankle.

Arthroscopy can confirm an injury to, and permit surgery on, the joint lining or a ligament or cartilage. It helps identify the cause of persistent pain or swelling and pinpoint why a joint has limited motion or is unstable or locking in one position. The examination can also reveal arthritis and any loose fragments of cartilage that are lying between the bones of the joint.

After you have been given an anesthetic and it has taken effect, the doctor makes a small cut in the skin and inserts a hollow tube with a central probe into the joint. The probe is removed and the end of the arthroscope is passed down the tube. Fluid is then introduced into the joint through a channel in the arthroscope to help separate the inner surfaces and give the doctor a good view.

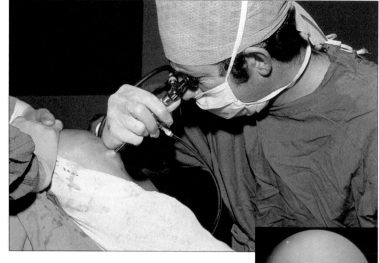

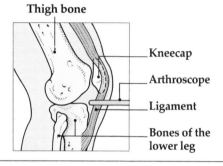

Thigh bone

Kneecap

Arthroscope

Ligament

Bones of the lower leg

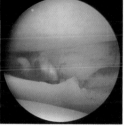

Damaged cartilage
This view of torn knee cartilage was taken through an arthroscope.

COLPOSCOPY

Colposcopy gives the doctor a detailed view of the cervix (neck of the uterus). The procedure is performed when a Pap smear has revealed abnormal cells. With the use of magnifying lenses, colposcopy shows any abnormal areas in the lining of the cervix and vagina.

How is the test done?

Colposcopy is a painless procedure. However, if a tissue sample (biopsy) is to be taken, a local anesthetic may be injected into the cervix to deaden the tissues so that you feel no discomfort.

After the doctor has performed a pelvic examination, he or she inserts a speculum into the vagina; in some cases, a diluted solution of acetic acid (household vinegar) may be swabbed on the cervix to clear it of mucus. The cervix and vagina are then viewed through the colposcope.

Position for colposcopy
For this examination, it is necessary to lie with your legs supported in stirrups in the position shown.

View of cervix
The red growths visible in the photograph at right are caused by keratosis, an overproduction of the skin protein keratin.

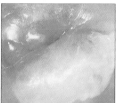

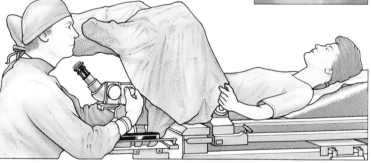

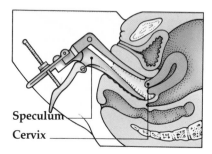

Speculum

Cervix

Examining the cervix
A speculum is inserted into the vagina to separate the walls widely (left). The doctor then uses the colposcope – a binocular instrument with a viewing head placed close to the entrance of the vagina – to view the cervix.

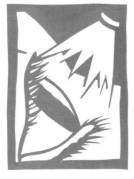

EYE EXAMINATIONS

NOWHERE IN MEDICINE is the use of projected light more valuable than in the diagnosis of eye disorders. The transparency of certain parts of the eye permits the ophthalmologist to employ a variety of specialized lamps and lenses to gain a detailed view of many of the delicate structures inside the eye.

Your ophthalmologist may examine your eyes for two different but sometimes related reasons – to assess the acuity of your vision or to diagnose and assess a disease before treatment. Eyes that are nearsighted, farsighted, or have an astigmatism (a defect of curvature in the corneas) are usually perfectly healthy. After your eyes have been tested, glasses or contact lenses are all that is required to restore normal vision.

If the ophthalmologist suspects that a disease is causing your symptoms, he or she will perform a variety of tests to establish its identity and severity.

The slit lamp
A slit-lamp examination is conducted using a binocular microscope linked to a powerful light source. The combination of magnification and light gives a detailed view of parts of the eye. The light beam can be adjusted and is often used in the form of a narrow, but intensely bright, vertical slit that can reveal abnormalities when directed at a section of the eye.

SLIT-LAMP EXAMINATION

Disorders studied using a slit lamp include corneal ulcers, inflammation in the eye, tumors of the iris, conjunctivitis, blood in the front chamber, cataracts, and opacities (clouding) in the vitreous fluid that fills the main cavity of the eye. The slit lamp also helps in locating foreign bodies and in assessing eye injuries.

How is the test done?
The ophthalmologist sits on one side of the slit lamp and you sit on the other, with your chin in a cup-shaped holder and your forehead rested against a flexible plastic strap. The examination is

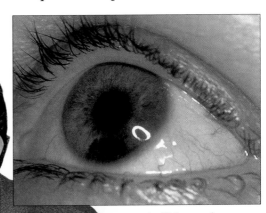

A slit-lamp view
The dark area seen under low-level magnification in the lower part of this iris is a suspected tumor.

usually done in semidarkness to increase the contrast between illuminated and nonilluminated areas and to highlight delicate detail of the eye structures.

Examining the retina

When the slit lamp is used to examine the retina, it may be necessary to neutralize the curve of the cornea by means of a contact lens. Your ophthalmologist will gently place a drop of a liquid local anesthetic onto each cornea to take away all sensation before he or she places the contact lens on your eye.

The slit lamp's high magnification helps identify many changes in the retina that may signify disease. Your ophthalmologist will also be able to see any minute abnormalities in the blood vessels of the retina and nerve fiber layers and any tiny holes in the retina.

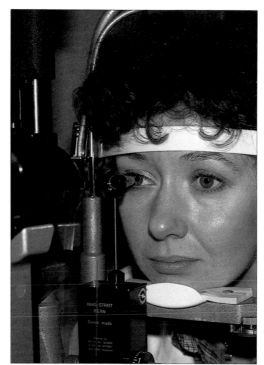

How the tonometer works
The tonometer is fitted to the slit lamp and has a small head with a flat, rounded end. Brought against the cornea of the eye, the tonometer causes a tiny area of flattening (applanation) in the center of your cornea. The ophthalmologist observes, through the tonometer head, a bright ring of fluorescein around the flattened area. When the pressure of the tonometer head on your eye is increased, the ring enlarges until it reaches a fixed standard. The force needed to achieve the standard degree of flattening is equal to the pressure inside your eye.

THE STRUCTURE OF THE EYE

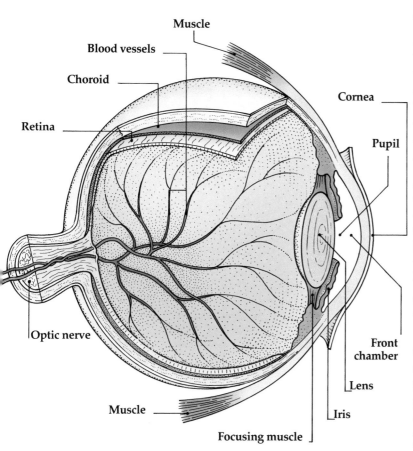

Muscle

Blood vessels

Choroid

Retina

Cornea

Pupil

Optic nerve

Front chamber

Lens

Muscle

Iris

Focusing muscle

APPLANATION TONOMETRY

Tonometry measures the pressure of the fluid within your eyes to ensure that it is within safe limits. High pressure within the eye can damage the optic nerve – a condition called glaucoma, which must be treated. People with glaucoma have tonometry performed at regular visits to their ophthalmologist to ensure that their treatment is still effective.

How is the test done?

After placing a drop of local anesthetic on both corneas, your ophthalmologist briefly touches each cornea with a tiny paper strip that has been impregnated with the orange dye fluorescein. This dye colors your tears and glows brightly when blue light is shined on it.

Sitting at the slit lamp, you will see a small circle of intense blue light coming steadily closer to one eye until you are unable to see anything else. After a second or two, the ophthalmologist will withdraw the light, and then examine your other eye in the same way.

79

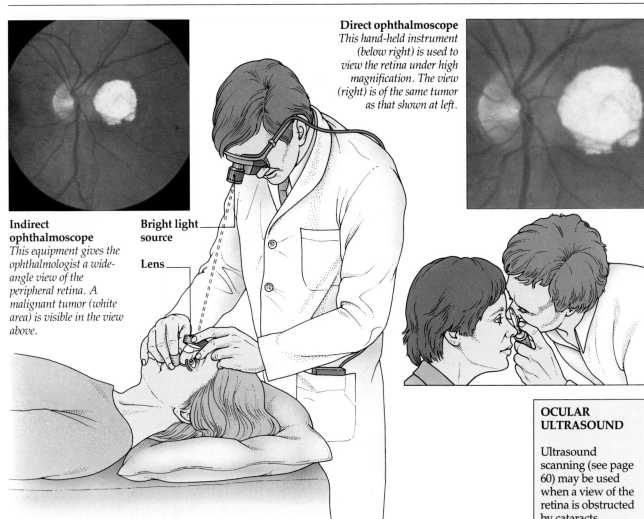

Indirect ophthalmoscope
This equipment gives the ophthalmologist a wide-angle view of the peripheral retina. A malignant tumor (white area) is visible in the view above.

Bright light source

Lens

Direct ophthalmoscope
This hand-held instrument (below right) is used to view the retina under high magnification. The view (right) is of the same tumor as that shown at left.

OCULAR ULTRASOUND

Ultrasound scanning (see page 60) may be used when a view of the retina is obstructed by cataracts, bleeding inside the eye, or opacity (clouding) of the cornea. Ultrasound-conducting jelly is first applied to the instrument head to form a seal. The transducer head is then applied to your closed eyelids. The operator views the ultrasound image on a screen and may take photographs, such as the one shown below.

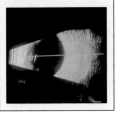

OPHTHALMOSCOPY

Although the slit lamp can provide high magnification of small areas of the retina, ophthalmoscopy is the standard examination for the inside of the back of the eye. The test can reveal retinal detachment, disease of the retina caused by diabetes or high blood pressure, degeneration of the retina, swelling or shrinking of the optic nerve, or a tumor in the layer under the retina. The formation of new blood vessels, and retinal tears, bleeding, and scarring – all associated with the advanced stages of diabetes – are also clearly visible.

How is the test done?
During a medical examination, any doctor may examine the retina with a hand-held direct ophthalmoscope. For a full examination by an ophthalmologist, your pupils are dilated (enlarged) with drops. When your pupils are fully dilated, you may be asked to recline in a darkened room.

On his or her head your ophthalmologist wears a binocular viewing instrument, fitted with a bright light source with which he or she illuminates the inside of your eye. A powerful hand-held lens is used to view a bright image of your retina. Although the light may seem painfully bright at first, your retinas will quickly adapt. There are no significant effects as a result of the bright light being directed into your eye.

If any abnormality is detected, it may be viewed under greater magnification, either with the slit lamp or with a direct ophthalmoscope.

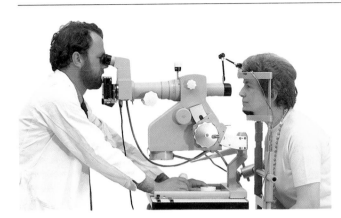

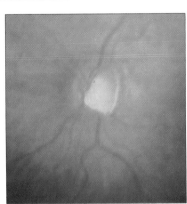

Photographing the retinal blood supply
In this test, the dye fluorescein is photographed under a blue light as it flows through the blood vessels of your retinas. Before the test begins, a color photograph (left) is taken of your retina.

FLUORESCEIN ANGIOGRAPHY

Fluorescein angiography is a test that reveals structural and disease-produced abnormalities in the blood vessels of the retina and choroid by introducing a fluorescent dye (fluorescein) into the blood vessels and then photographing them. Abnormalities that can be seen include new vessel formation, which may threaten sight; abnormal leakage of dye, indicating abnormal vessel function; and areas of the retina showing no fluorescence, an indication that they may not be receiving blood. This test helps the diagnosis of conditions affecting not only the retina but also the blood vessel-filled choroid layer beneath it. Conditions diagnosed by fluorescein angiography include diabetic retinal disease, inflammation of the blood vessels, and degeneration of the macula, the site on the retina of greatest visual acuity.

How is the test done?

Your pupils are first dilated with drops, and color photographs of the retina are made. The camera is then reloaded with a fine-grain black and white film, which shows the detail of the fluorescein glow.

At this point you will be given an injection of a sterile solution of fluorescein into a vein. A rapid succession of retinal photographs are then taken as the dye first moves through the retinal arteries, then through the delicate capillaries, and finally through the veins.

RETINAL CIRCULATION SEEN BY ANGIOGRAPHY

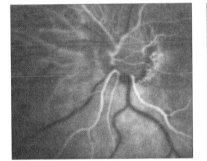

1 The dye fluorescein is making its first appearance, lightening the retinal arteries.

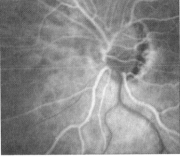

2 The arterial branches are filling with dye, revealing the full arterial network.

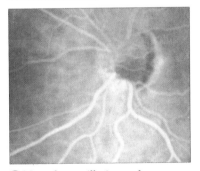

3 Now the capillaries and formerly dark veins are beginning to fill with fluorescein dye.

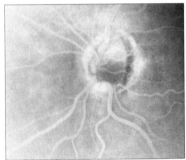

4 The capillaries and veins are flooded; at this moment the maximum dye is visible.

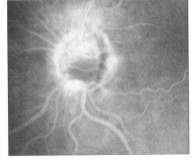

5 There is very little dye in the artery, and the veins and capillaries are emptying.

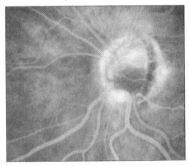

6 The dye is now diluted and has largely flowed out of arteries, capillary beds, and veins.

ELECTRICAL TESTS

ELECTRICAL ACTIVITY in nerve and muscle cells occurs as a result of the flow of ions (electrically charged particles) between the inside and outside of the cell membrane. Electricity is vital to the functioning of the brain, nerves, and muscles, including the heart. Because the body conducts electricity, electrical changes can be detected on the body's surface by a sensitive instrument. There are specific changes in these electrical patterns when certain disorders are present.

Electrocardiography (the measurement of electrical activity in the heart) and electroencephalography (the measurement of electrical activity in the brain) are among the most frequently used electrical tests. Other, much less commonly used tests include evoked responses (the measurement of electrical activity in the brain or spinal cord or in a nerve in response to stimulation) and electromyography (the measurement of electrical activity in the muscles).

Having an ECG
Electrocardiography is carried out by attaching electrodes to the arms, legs, and chest. The electrical impulses picked up by the electrodes travel through wires to a recording machine, which produces an image on paper or on a screen. During the procedure you are asked to lie still, relax, and breathe normally. If you move or talk, the tracing can be distorted.

ELECTROCARDIOGRAPHY

The heart is a strong muscle that pumps blood to the lungs and the rest of the body by contracting and relaxing in a regular pattern. The signals that tell the muscle to contract come from the sinoatrial node, the heart's pacemaker, and are carried from one part of the heart

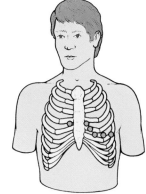

Placement of electrodes
The chest lead may be moved to any of six points on the chest so that electrical activity in different parts of the heart can be detected.

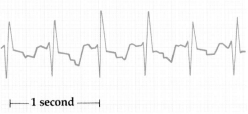

|—— 1 second ——|

Abnormal heartbeat
This ECG shows that the patient has atrial tachycardia, in which the upper heart chambers (atria) beat more rapidly than the ventricles. Six heartbeats are represented on the tracing.

READING AN ELECTROCARDIOGRAM

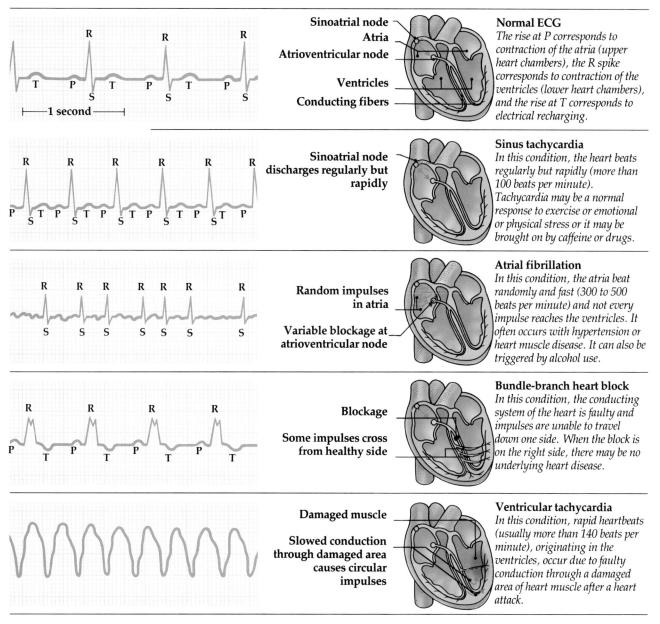

Normal ECG
The rise at P corresponds to contraction of the atria (upper heart chambers), the R spike corresponds to contraction of the ventricles (lower heart chambers), and the rise at T corresponds to electrical recharging.

Sinoatrial node discharges regularly but rapidly

Sinus tachycardia
In this condition, the heart beats regularly but rapidly (more than 100 beats per minute). Tachycardia may be a normal response to exercise or emotional or physical stress or it may be brought on by caffeine or drugs.

Random impulses in atria

Variable blockage at atrioventricular node

Atrial fibrillation
In this condition, the atria beat randomly and fast (300 to 500 beats per minute) and not every impulse reaches the ventricles. It often occurs with hypertension or heart muscle disease. It can also be triggered by alcohol use.

Blockage

Some impulses cross from healthy side

Bundle-branch heart block
In this condition, the conducting system of the heart is faulty and impulses are unable to travel down one side. When the block is on the right side, there may be no underlying heart disease.

Damaged muscle

Slowed conduction through damaged area causes circular impulses

Ventricular tachycardia
In this condition, rapid heartbeats (usually more than 140 beats per minute), originating in the ventricles, occur due to faulty conduction through a damaged area of heart muscle after a heart attack.

to another by electrical impulses. These electrical impulses are detected and recorded in electrocardiography. The image produced during the test is called an electrocardiogram (ECG). It shows any abnormalities in the heart's rate or rhythm and is useful for diagnosing disorders and monitoring treatment.

Diagnostic uses

If you have experienced chest pain, breathlessness, dizziness, palpitations, or fainting attacks, your doctor may arrange for you to have an ECG. The test can show signs of coronary heart disease, heart attack, arrhythmia (disturbances of heart rhythm), and a variety of other heart disorders. An ECG can also identify abnormal levels of certain minerals in the blood that control electrical activity in the heart. If you are being treated with medication for a heart disorder, an ECG may be suggested to keep track of the safety and effectiveness of your treatment. In other cases, a physical examination may include an ECG.

Normal and abnormal heartbeats
The heart at rest beats at a regular rate of 60 to 100 beats per minute in adults. Electrical impulses originate in the sinoatrial node, travel through the atria, causing contraction, and reach the atrioventricular node. They then travel via conducting fibers to the ventricles, which also contract. An abnormal heartbeat may be too fast, too slow, or irregular.

An ECG is ordinarily taken while you are at rest. If your symptoms are brought on by exercise, the ECG may be performed while you engage in vigorous physical activity, usually while walking on a treadmill or riding an exercise bicycle. An abnormal pattern of electrical activity during exercise may indicate that you have coronary heart disease or a congenital heart disorder. More tests, such as thallium scanning, PET scanning, or angiography, may be used to determine the extent of the disease.

If symptoms such as palpitations, chest pain, fainting, or dizziness come on intermittently and last for only a short time, you may have ambulatory electrocardiography, also called Holter monitoring, in which a continuous, 24-hour recording is made while you go about your daily activities.

Exercise ECG
In this test, you walk on a treadmill that is gradually adjusted to make you work harder. Your condition is monitored continuously and the test is stopped immediately if your blood pressure falls, the ECG tracing becomes abnormal, or such symptoms as chest pains, palpitations, or breathlessness develop. Monitoring is continued for at least 5 minutes after you stop walking on the treadmill.

Blood pressure cuff

Electrodes

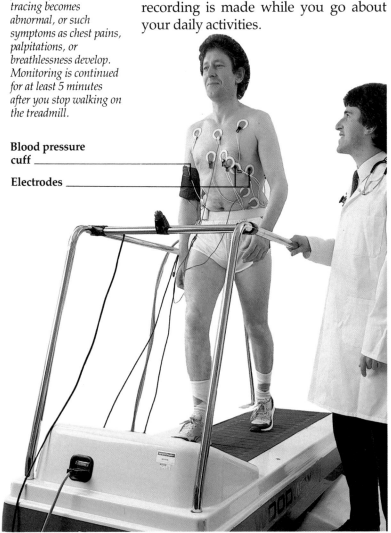

Preparing for the test

You may be advised not to smoke or consume any caffeine or alcohol for 24 hours before the test. You should tell your doctor if you are taking any medication, because some drugs alter the electrical activity in the heart.

Before the electrodes are attached, your skin is cleaned with alcohol. In some people, the chest is shaved. The skin may also be gently roughed up to improve the pickup of electrical impulses. A conducting jelly is then used to apply the suction cups to the skin.

After the test

When the test is over, the electrodes are removed and the conducting jelly is wiped off your skin with a damp cloth. Your doctor may discuss the results with you or ask you to return for another appointment. After an ambulatory ECG, a computer assists in analyzing the recording for any abnormalities. Whatever type of ECG you have, more tests may be required to confirm a diagnosis.

Are there any risks?

Resting and ambulatory ECGs are completely safe. In very rare cases, the exertion required for an exercise ECG may provoke severe chest pain, a heart attack, or cardiac arrest (heart stoppage), which is why the test is carefully supervised by a doctor with all the necessary resuscitation equipment nearby.

Ambulatory ECG   **Tape recorder**
For this test, you wear a portable recorder (called a Holter monitor) that makes a continuous recording. You continue your daily activities, keeping a log of everything you do and noting any symptoms you have. Sometimes you are given a monitor that you can activate yourself, so that you can make a recording whenever you feel symptoms.

CASE HISTORY
DIZZY SPELLS AND BLACKOUTS

ELLEN HAD BEEN **suffering from attacks of dizziness for 2 months. At first, she thought that the dizzy spells were occurring because she had been upset since moving from her old family home. She realized that she hadn't been her usual cheerful self since the move. Ellen collapsed suddenly in the kitchen one morning and was rushed to the local hospital.**

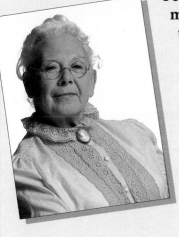

PERSONAL DETAILS
Name Ellen Brown
Age 81
Occupation Retired music teacher
Family Ellen's parents both died in their 70s, her father of a stroke and her mother after a heart attack. Ellen lives with her daughter, who is in good health.

MEDICAL BACKGROUND
Ellen has arthritis, which makes it difficult to climb stairs. Otherwise, her health has been good.

THE CONSULTATION
When Ellen arrives in the emergency room, she is fully conscious but confused. She manages to tell the doctor about the dizzy spells but says that she has never blacked out before. The doctor examines Ellen and finds that her pulse rate is only 30 beats per minute (well below the normal of about 70 beats per minute) and her blood pressure is low.

FURTHER INVESTIGATION
The doctor decides to perform an immediate electrocardiogram (ECG) to identify the source of the slow rhythm in Ellen's heart. Electrodes are attached to Ellen's wrists, ankles, and chest, and the ECG machine is turned on.

The tracing shows an obvious abnormality – the "spikes" in the tracing, which correspond to the contractions of Ellen's ventricles (lower chambers of her heart), do not follow regularly in sequence after the "blips" corresponding to contractions of the atria (upper chambers). Instead, the atria and ventricles appear to be contracting independently of each other. The ventricles are also contracting at a much slower than normal rate.

THE DIAGNOSIS
From the ECG trace, the doctor concludes that the cause of Ellen's dizzy spells and the blackout is complete HEART BLOCK. In a healthy heart, electrical waves pass regularly from the atria to the ventricles of the heart, so that they contract in sequence. However, in Ellen's heart, there is a block to the transmission of the waves, so the ventricles have taken up their own, much slower, rate of contraction. Because of this, the flow of blood to Ellen's brain has been reduced, which explains her dizziness and blackout.

Ellen's heart block may be the result of a minor heart attack that passed unnoticed but that caused the conduction pathway in her heart muscle to be damaged.

THE TREATMENT
Ellen's doctor inserts a pacemaker to get her heart beating properly again.

In less than 24 hours, she feels much better and goes home. With her heart now being paced at 70 beats per minute, she suffers no more dizzy spells and is able to lead a normal, active life.

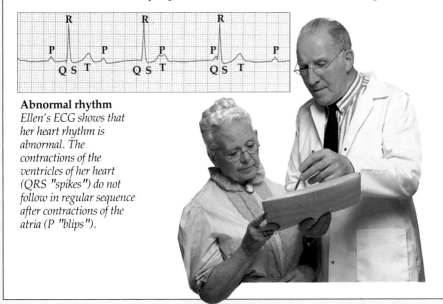

Abnormal rhythm
Ellen's ECG shows that her heart rhythm is abnormal. The contractions of the ventricles of her heart (QRS "spikes") do not follow in regular sequence after contractions of the atria (P "blips").

ELECTRO-ENCEPHALOGRAPHY

The brain produces tiny amounts of electricity that can be detected by electrodes attached to the scalp. The electrical impulses picked up by the electrodes are conveyed through wires to an electroencephalograph, which amplifies the impulses a million times and records them as a tracing on paper (called an electroencephalogram or EEG). The types of waves recorded on the tracing are classified by letters of the Greek alphabet (alpha, beta, theta, delta, and so on) based on their frequency. Normal patterns differ depending on the age of the patient and his or her state of wakefulness. Certain waves indicate the presence of different types of epilepsy.

Why is it done?

An EEG is used primarily to diagnose epilepsy (and to determine its type) and, in modified form, to investigate sleep disorders. It is occasionally used to help diagnose encephalitis and meningitis (inflammation of the brain and the membranes that cover the brain) or to evaluate the extent of brain damage after a stroke, although computed tomography (CT) scanning or magnetic resonance imaging (MRI) is usually preferred for this purpose. An EEG helps determine brain death in some states.

An EEG cannot indicate a person's mental ability or diagnose psychiatric disorders such as schizophrenia.

Preparing for the procedure

Tranquilizers and sedatives are sometimes withheld for 24 to 48 hours before the test, and you are asked not to consume any caffeine for several hours before the procedure. Just before the EEG, you should eat a small meal. If the test is performed on an empty stomach, the resulting low blood sugar levels can produce abnormal results. It is not necessary for your hair to be cut.

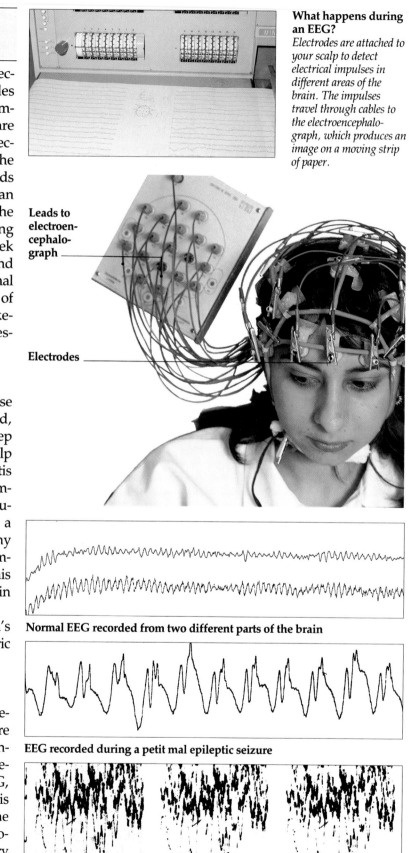

What happens during an EEG?
Electrodes are attached to your scalp to detect electrical impulses in different areas of the brain. The impulses travel through cables to the electroencephalograph, which produces an image on a moving strip of paper.

Leads to electroencephalograph

Electrodes

Normal EEG recorded from two different parts of the brain

EEG recorded during a petit mal epileptic seizure

EEG recorded during grand mal epileptic seizure

Having an EEG

The test is carried out in a room that is isolated from outside electrical activity. You either sit in a reclining chair or lie down on a bed. You may be given a mild sedative so that you are not restless during the examination. Sixteen or more electrodes are attached to the scalp, usually with special conducting jelly and a harmless, removable paste. Sometimes, tiny needle electrodes are inserted into the scalp, a procedure that is not painful because the scalp has very few nerve endings. Once the electrodes are in position, recordings are made with your eyes closed and then open. During the recordings, you will be asked to move and talk as little as possible because doing so interferes with the EEG. Sometimes a recording is taken while you sleep. The test lasts about an hour.

After the test

A nurse will help you remove the electrode jelly and paste from your hair. Your doctor may want to discuss the results of the test with you immediately or may ask you to return for an appointment several days later.

WHAT ARE THE RISKS OF EEG?

In rare cases, people prone to epilepsy have a seizure during the test, especially if any anticonvulsant medication being taken has temporarily been stopped. If a seizure occurs, the doctor and nurse will give the necessary treatment.

EEG for sleep disorder
If you are being tested for a sleep problem, an EEG may be performed. You will be asked not to sleep at all the night before and, if necessary, your doctor will give you a sedative to help you sleep during the test.

ASK YOUR DOCTOR
ELECTRICAL TESTS

Q **My husband's doctor wants him to have some evoked response studies. How are these tests done and what are they for?**

A For auditory, brain stem, or visual evoked response studies, electrodes will be attached to your husband's scalp to measure changes in the brain's electrical activity in response to stimulation of the eye or ear. The tests are painless and provide useful information about the pathways within your husband's nervous system.

Q **I recently had an EEG. At times during the test I was asked to breathe deeply and rapidly. I also had a strobe light flashed in front of my eyes. Why was this?**

A Breathing heavily affects blood chemistry, which causes changes in the electrical activity in the brain. These changes, detectable on an EEG, may indicate a tendency to epilepsy or may help in the diagnosis of epilepsy. A strobe light also produces changes in electrical brain activity that can have similar diagnostic significance.

Q **My father died of a heart attack, and I am worried that I might have inherited a tendency to heart disease. Should I have an ECG?**

A Measuring the level of cholesterol and other fats in the blood would be a more useful approach. Heart disease that runs in families is most often due to an inherited tendency to a high level of cholesterol in the blood. Much more rarely there is a structural or electrical abnormality. An ECG rarely shows abnormalities in someone who does not have symptoms of heart disease. An exercise ECG might be more helpful.

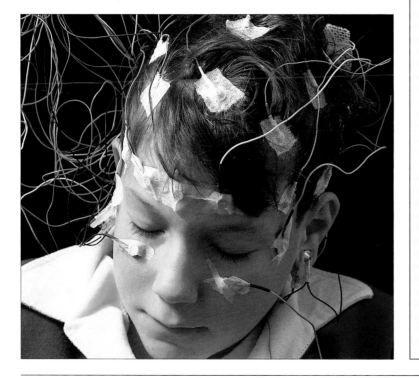

HEARING TESTS

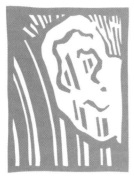

HEARING IS ONE of your most precious senses – perhaps almost as important as sight. But people are often reluctant to admit they have a hearing problem. In other cases, friends or loved ones don't realize they are having trouble hearing until someone tells them. Most forms of hearing loss are treatable by surgery or a hearing aid. If you are not hearing well or someone in your family does not seem to be responding to sound in the usual way, consult your doctor.

Having audiometry
For audiometric tests, you sit in a small, soundproof room with glass windows. You wear earphones, through which sounds are transmitted to one ear at a time. The loudness at which you are able to hear each sound is noted (in decibels) and marked on a chart called an audiogram.

Hearing tests determine how well you can hear sounds of varying frequency (pitch) and intensity (loudness). They can also help determine whether a hearing aid would be effective and, if so, what type would be most beneficial.

Sensorineural hearing loss
This audiogram shows the hearing thresholds of a person with sensorineural hearing loss. Air conduction (circles) and bone conduction (arrows) hearing are diminished, particularly at high frequencies.

DIAGNOSTIC USES

Hearing tests help the doctor establish the extent and pattern of any hearing loss. They can also determine what type

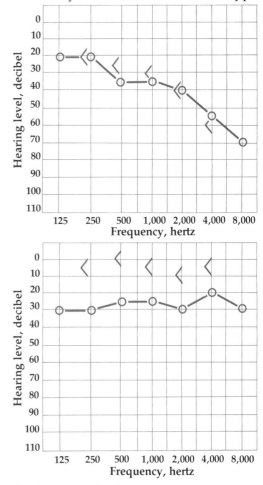

Conductive hearing loss
In this defect, air conduction hearing levels (circles) are diminished but bone conduction hearing levels (arrows) are normal across the range of frequencies.

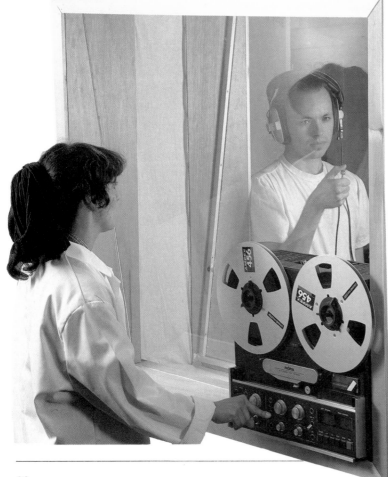

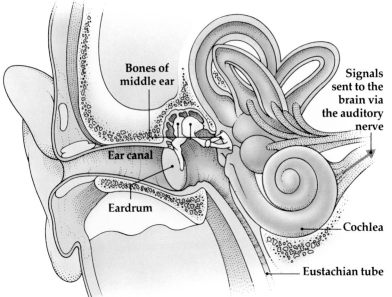

How we hear
Sound waves entering the outer-ear canal cause the eardrum to vibrate. These vibrations are transmitted by the bones of the middle ear to the cochlea, which turns them into electrical signals and sends them to the brain.

When are tests performed?

Hearing tests are often given to children as part of a general assessment of their development. They are also performed when a person is having difficulty hearing and when someone is suspected of having hearing loss (such as a child who is slow in learning to talk or an older person who is confused). People who are exposed to loud noise at work also should have regular tests to be sure no damage has occurred.

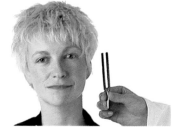

of hearing loss you have by comparing how well you hear when a sound source is placed near the outer-ear canal (air conduction) and when it is held against the skull (bone conduction).

If air conduction hearing is diminished but bone conduction hearing is normal, you have conductive hearing loss – a problem in the transmission of sound through the outer-ear canal and the middle ear. If both air conduction hearing and bone conduction hearing are diminished, you have sensorineural deafness. This means there is damage to the cochlea in the inner ear, to the nerves that connect the ear to the brain, or to the hearing centers in the brain itself.

Types of hearing tests

In the simplest type of hearing test, a tuning fork is used to determine whether hearing loss is conductive or sensorineural. More sophisticated tests, known as audiometry, involve the use of an audiometer, an instrument that can accurately produce sounds that span a range of frequencies and intensities within the capabilities of human hearing.

Weber's test
In this procedure, which helps diagnose unilateral hearing defects, a vibrating tuning fork is placed against the forehead. In conductive hearing loss, the sound is heard better in the ear with the poorer hearing because that ear is undisturbed by external sounds in the environment.

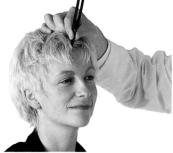

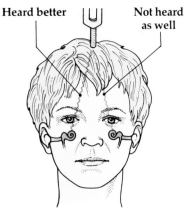

Conductive deafness in right ear

Rinne's test
A vibrating tuning fork is placed near the outer-ear canal (for air conduction) and then against the mastoid bone (for bone conduction). In a normal ear or one with sensorineural hearing loss, air conduction is better than bone conduction. In conductive hearing loss, bone conduction is better.

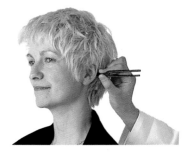

Normal hearing or sensorineural hearing loss in left ear

IMPEDANCE AUDIOMETRY TEST

This type of test is used to determine whether middle-ear damage is causing your hearing loss and what type of middle-ear problem there is.

You will have a probe fitted snugly into your outer-ear canal to seal it off from outside pressure and sound. The probe emits a continuous sound while air is pumped through it at varying pressures. A microphone in the probe registers the different patterns of sounds that are reflected back from the eardrum as the pressure changes. The patterns, which are recorded on a graph called a tympanogram, indicate whether the eardrum and the bones in the middle ear are moving normally. The device can also be used to measure air pressure in the middle ear. In a healthy person, the pressure on both sides of the eardrum remains equal. Blockage of the eustachian tube, fluid in the middle ear, or a perforated eardrum produce characteristic patterns on the tympanogram.

Microphone

Electronic tone generator

Air pump and pressure meter

Ear canal

Inner ear

Eardrum   Middle ear

Fitting the probe
The probe used for impedance audiometry must fit closely in the outer-ear canal if the procedure is to work effectively. A cuff of an appropriate size is chosen and attached to the probe to achieve this. If necessary, some silicone putty is used to ensure an airtight seal.

AUDIOMETRY

For this test, you are asked to put on large, padded earphones, which are connected to the audiometer outside the soundproof room. Sounds are transmitted through one ear at a time, while the other ear is prevented from hearing them. The sound frequency is increased in stages from 250 to 8,000 hertz (cycles per second). For each frequency the volume is gradually increased until you signal that you can hear it. Alternatively, the test may start with a loud sound, which is gradually decreased in intensity. The intensity at which you hear each frequency is recorded.

The test is repeated with sounds transmitted through a plastic oscillator held against your mastoid bone by a head-band. This procedure tests your bone conduction hearing.

To test a person who may not be able to respond when a sound is heard (for example, an infant), electrodes can be placed on the scalp to detect changes in brain activity that occur in response to different sounds. This technique is called evoked response audiometry.

Impedance audiometry tests may be used to obtain more information about the cause of hearing loss (see box above).

Speech audiometry

To test your ability to recognize spoken words, the audiometer is used to present a succession of two-syllable words at varying intensities. The intensity at which you can correctly repeat 50 percent of the words, known as the speech threshold, is recorded. The words are then played again at a level of 40 decibels above the speech threshold, and the number you hear correctly is recorded and converted into a percentage. The normal score is 90 to 100 percent. A person who has conductive hearing loss can still achieve this score. A person who has sensorineural hearing loss may have a substantially reduced score.

Results

The doctor will discuss the results of the tests with you and, if treatment is required, will advise you on the benefits of surgery or a hearing aid. Many people with conductive hearing loss can be completely cured by surgery; others adapt well to hearing aids. Sensorineural hearing loss may be slightly more difficult to treat. However, recent technological advances have resulted in hearing aids to suit most needs.

How well can you understand speech?
To test your ability to understand speech, you may be asked to sit in a quiet room while a series of recorded words are played through headphones. You will be asked to repeat as many words as you can. The number of words you hear correctly is noted and an assessment is made.

Classifying word recognition ability
Your ability to recognize spoken words is classified according to the percentage of words (played to you through headphones) you are able to repeat correctly.

Excellent	90 to 100 percent correct
Good	75 to 90 percent correct
Fair	60 to 75 percent correct
Poor	40 to 60 percent correct
Very poor	0 to 40 percent correct

ASK YOUR DOCTOR
HEARING TESTS

Q During audiometry tests I had recently, a strange hissing noise was sometimes played through the earphones into one ear while the other ear was being tested. Why?

A When sounds are played into one ear, they sometimes travel through the bones of the skull to the other ear. This may distort the results of the test. Playing sounds of all frequencies, called white noise, into the ear not being tested masks any sounds conducted through bone.

Q I am going for a hearing test next week. Are any special preparations required?

A You don't have to do anything special before a hearing test. However, if you have been exposed to very loud noises (loud enough to cause ringing in your ears or to make conversation difficult) within the past 16 hours, the test will be postponed. Before the test, the doctor will examine your ears with an otoscope (a viewing instrument) to ensure they are not blocked by wax.

Q I suffer from ringing in my ears. Would it be helpful for me to have a hearing test?

A Yes. You need to have the cause of the ringing in your ears, or tinnitus, identified. Most often, tinnitus is due to hearing loss caused by noise exposure or from the progressive loss of hearing that occurs with age. Tinnitus, especially if it is one-sided, may in rare cases be the first sign of acoustic neuroma, a curable tumor. When tinnitus is associated with attacks of dizziness or vomiting, it is usually due to a condition called Meniere's disease, a degeneration of the inner ear.

CHAPTER FIVE

BODY FLUID AND TISSUE ANALYSIS

EVERY YEAR, several billion medical laboratory tests are performed in the US – an estimated 20 to 30 tests per person. Most of these are blood tests, but samples of urine, sputum, numerous other body fluids, and tissue are also taken and sent to a laboratory for analysis. This chapter looks at how and why these tests are performed and how they can help your doctor establish or confirm a diagnosis. The first section explains how doctors obtain different samples for analysis. Most people know how a blood sample is taken, but what about a nasopharyngeal swab, a needle biopsy of the liver, or aspiration of fluid from a knee or elbow joint? In most cases, these procedures are not as uncomfortable as you might imagine. The remaining sections of this chapter describe what happens to the samples when they reach the laboratory. The sec-

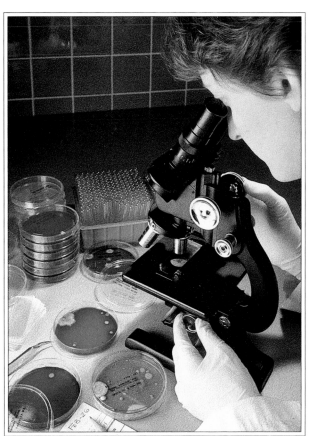

tion on whole blood tests covers hematology, which is concerned primarily with the number, size, shape, and functioning of blood cells. Hematology is used principally to diagnose diseases of blood cell production, notably anemia and leukemia, and various types of bleeding disorders. In addition, hematological findings can help your doctor diagnose many other disorders. The following section, on chemi-

cal and immunological tests, covers the areas of chemical pathology (the use of chemical analysis of a body fluid sample to look for signs of disease) and immunology, in which the body's immune system is examined for evidence of infectious disease or immune system disorders, such as allergy. The final section, on culturing techniques and microscopy, is an introduction to microbiology, cytopathology, and histopathology. In medicine, microbiology is primarily concerned with identifying agents of infectious disease, such as bacteria and fungi, under the microscope or growing them on culture plates. Cytopathology and histopathology are the microscopic examinations of body cells and thin slices of tissue to find changes in shape, structure, or appearance that are characteristic of disease. These examinations are among the most precise and important diagnostic methods. The last 20 years have brought a large increase in the number and sophistication of laboratory tests; many doctors themselves may find it challenging to keep up with what tests are available. In this chapter, there is room to mention only some of the most important methods, but the A-Z OF MEDICAL TESTS on pages 128 to 141 describes more than one hundred additional tests.

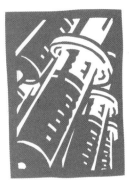

HOW SAMPLES ARE TAKEN

L ABORATORY ANALYSIS or microscopic examination of samples of your blood, urine, and many other body fluids and tissues is invaluable in confirming the cause of disease. The manner in which these samples are taken must be carefully controlled, however, if the tests are to give an accurate indication of your condition.

Whatever type of sample your doctor requires from you, it must fulfill two criteria to be of optimum value in the laboratory. First, it must be fresh enough not to have lost its distinctive characteristics. Second, it must not be contaminated with any substance that may affect the accuracy of the laboratory results.

BLOOD SAMPLES

A sample of your blood may be subjected to a wide range of tests. The tests check the state of the blood cells and determine the levels of a wide range of biochemical substances in the serum (the clear fluid

HOW A BLOOD SAMPLE IS TAKEN

Making the vein prominent
A soft band is wrapped around the upper arm. The band does not interfere with the flow of blood into your arm through the main artery, but does constrict the veins so that they stand up prominently.

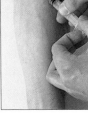

Inserting the needle
After the selected site has been cleaned with alcohol (above), the needle is inserted just under the skin, parallel to the vein and a small distance away from it (left). This causes little or no sensation.

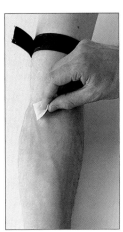

Taking the sample
The needle point is brought over the vein and allowed to pass through it. The piston of the syringe is pulled back, creating a vacuum that is filled by the required amount of blood.

that separates from blood when it clots). Plasma (the clear fluid that remains if the blood cells are removed) is also used for certain biochemical tests. In addition, blood may be taken so that any infectious organisms can be cultured from it.

How is the sample taken?

Some tests require only a drop or two of blood, in which case a fingertip puncture with a sterile, surgical knife (a lancet) is sufficient. If more blood is required, it is usually taken from a vein at the bend of your elbow, using a hollow needle attached to either a sterile disposable syringe or to a vacuum device.

The nurse or technician first makes the vein prominent by wrapping a soft tube or band around your upper arm to act as a tourniquet. The skin over your vein is then cleaned with alcohol and the needle is inserted. The piston in the syringe is then drawn back (or the vacuum seal is broken when the rubber cap of the collecting tube is punctured by the base of the needle) and the required amount of blood is drawn.

In rare cases, it is necessary to take blood from an artery. The walls of arteries are sensitive and an injection of a local anesthetic may be needed.

URINE SAMPLES

Your urine provides important information about several systems in your body. Many tests are done on urine in the laboratory, but your doctor can perform several tests in his or her office by using special test strips that have been impregnated with a range of chemicals. These strips are dipped into the urine sample to confirm whether or not the person being tested has a particular abnormality. The presence of sugar or acetone and other ketones can signify diabetes, protein can indicate some types of kidney disease, and blood in the urine sample suggests a variety of disorders of the kidneys, ureters, or bladder.

TESTING URINE FOR ABNORMALITIES

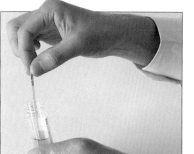

Dipping the strip
First, the strip is dipped into the urine sample. Dip-test strips vary according to the manufacturer, both in their chemical constituents and in the timing of the test. The strip shown here tests the urine for the presence of protein.

Interpreting the results
Any excess urine is shaken from the strip and then the timing begins. When the specified period has elapsed, the color of the strip is compared against a printed chart.

How is the sample taken?

Providing a urine sample is a simple process. If infection is suspected, you may be asked to provide a midstream specimen early one morning after you awaken. Otherwise, your doctor may give you a container and ask you to pass a sample of urine in the washroom.

To provide a midstream specimen, first pass some urine, then collect a small quantity in a thoroughly cleaned wide-necked container or conical urine glass. Urine in the bladder is normally sterile and may become contaminated as it is being passed. For this reason, uncircumcised men should pull back the foreskin and wash the end of the penis with soap and water before urinating. Women should wash the genital area.

FECAL SAMPLES

The appearance of a fecal sample can tell your doctor a great deal about your health. Clay-colored feces indicate that bile pigments are not getting into the intestine from the liver and suggest an obstruction of the bile ducts. Fatty stools that are frothy, that float, and are particularly foul-smelling suggest an intestinal disorder. Bright red blood in the feces indicates bleeding from hemorrhoids or from somewhere low in the large intestine or rectum. A tar-black appearance is a sign of bleeding higher in the upper gastrointestinal tract or in the upper part of the large intestine. There may be excessive mucus in colitis and other conditions, or pus if the lower bowel is infected. Your doctor can obtain more diagnostic information from chemical tests and microscopic examination of fecal samples performed in the laboratory.

How is the sample taken?

An amount of feces the size of a walnut is sufficient for a sample. You should defecate into a clean, dry receptacle, such as a bedpan or a child's potty, and then transfer a small quantity into a container. Your doctor probably will give you a container with a spoon fixed to the inside of the lid for this purpose. Try to avoid contaminating the feces with urine. The sample is then sent to the laboratory as soon as possible for examination.

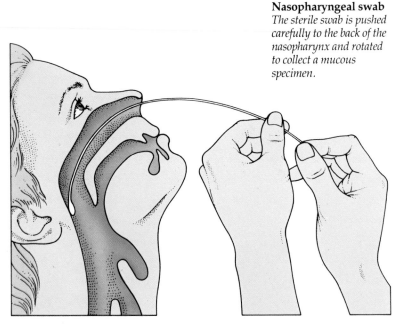

Nasopharyngeal swab
The sterile swab is pushed carefully to the back of the nasopharynx and rotated to collect a mucous specimen.

SPUTUM SAMPLES

A sample of coughed-up sputum (not spit-out saliva) may be required for culturing, microscopic examination, and bacteriological analysis. Your doctor will give you a cup in which to provide the sample. Diagnosis of pneumonia or tuberculosis can be confirmed if certain bacteria are identified.

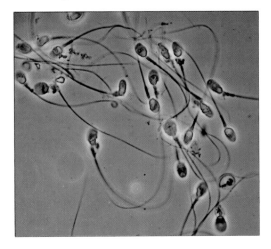

Semen samples
Semen samples are needed to test male fertility and to see if a vasectomy has been successful. The samples are examined for mobility of the sperm. The sperm are also counted. Since the sample must be analyzed within 2 hours, it is obtained by masturbation at the doctor's office or clinic.

BACTERIAL SWAB

Whenever a bacterial infection is considered a likely cause of a health problem, it is common to take a specimen from the affected part of the body for analysis. This is done quickly with a sterile, cotton-tipped swab that is immediately placed in a culture tube containing nutrients. The nutrients ensure that the bacteria do not die on the way to the laboratory. Your doctor makes sure that the swab touches only the tissue, discharge, or other area under investigation, to avoid other contamination.

How is the sample taken?

All bacterial swabs are done in much the same way. For a throat swab, the doctor holds your tongue down with a tongue depressor and then gently rubs the swab across the area of your tonsils. For a conjunctival swab, which may be done to confirm suspected conjunctivitis, you will be asked to look upward. While the lower eyelid is pulled slightly away from the eye, the swab is gently moved along the membrane that lines the inside of your lower lid. Nasal swabs are taken from the mucous membrane that lines the inside of your nostrils.

GASTRIC SAMPLES

The examination of samples of gastric juice taken from the stomach can assist in the diagnosis of several disorders of the digestive tract. Absence of acid in the juice, especially after the injection of the acid-stimulating drug pentagastrin, is an indication of pernicious anemia or stomach cancer. Too much acid, on the other hand, may be caused by a tumor of the pancreas. Samples of gastric juice are also taken before and after a vagotomy, an operation in which the acid-stimulating nerves of the stomach are cut, to test the operation's effectiveness.

How is the sample taken?

Gastric juice is collected via a soft rubber or plastic tube that is passed into your stomach via your mouth or nose. The lubricated tube passes down easily if you swallow continuously while it is being guided; after a short time you will not be aware of the tube in your throat.

Once the end of the tube has reached your stomach, a syringe is attached and a sample of gastric fluid is drawn up the tube and placed in a sterile container for analysis at a laboratory.

CERVICAL (PAP) SMEAR

The cervical smear, or Pap test, is a well-known screening test for early signs of cancer of the cervix (neck of the uterus). This cancer is completely curable if detected at the stage known as carcinoma in situ, in which cancerous changes in the cells of the cervix have begun, but have not penetrated the surface. Earlier precancerous changes, called dysplasia, can also be detected and treated.

How is the sample taken?

The purpose of a Pap smear is to take a sample of cells from your cervical opening for analysis. You lie on your back with your knees raised and apart, with a sheet covering the lower half of your

PERFORMING A PAP SMEAR

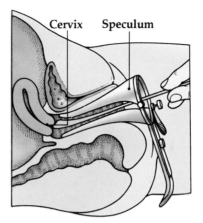

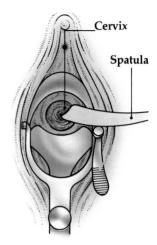

Exposing the cervix
An instrument called a speculum is used to separate the vaginal walls, allowing access to the cervix.

Taking the sample
A spatula is passed through the speculum and is used to scrape cells from the cervical canal.

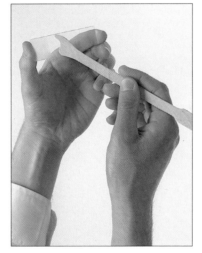

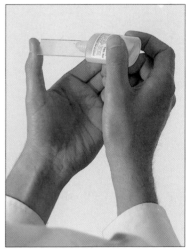

Preparing the slide
The spatula is carefully withdrawn and the tissue sample is smeared onto a glass slide.

Fixing the sample
The slide is immediately immersed in a fixative solution (or sprayed with a fixative) and sent to the laboratory.

body. The gynecologist then gently inserts a speculum, separating the walls of the vagina to expose the cervix. If you remain relaxed, the procedure causes no pain or discomfort. A small spatula is used to scrape some cells from the cervix. These cells are smeared onto a microscope slide, stained, and sent for examination. Any abnormal cells are apparent to the cytotechnician or mechanical cell analyzer viewing the smear.

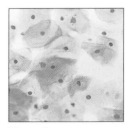

Normal smear
In this microscopic view of a Pap smear, the cervical cells are healthy and there is no abnormality.

CASE HISTORY
AN ABNORMAL PAP SMEAR

LISA HAS NOT SEEN **her gynecologist for 3 years. Several months ago, she received a letter from her doctor's office reminding her she was due to have another cervical (Pap) smear, but she ignored it. Two years ago, she and her husband were divorced, and she has not had a sexual relationship since then. She was prompted to make an appointment for a Pap smear after reading an article in a magazine.**

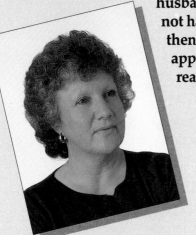

PERSONAL DETAILS
Name Lisa Costello
Age 49
Occupation Cosmetologist
Family Father died of a heart attack 5 years ago. Mother is in good health.

MEDICAL BACKGROUND
Lisa has an obstetric history of five pregnancies, with three normal deliveries and two miscarriages. She has taken contraceptive pills intermittently for 15 years and has had regular pelvic examinations during that time. She was prescribed antidepressants for 3 months after her divorce, but has not needed medication since then.

THE CONSULTATION
Lisa tells her gynecologist that she would like to have a Pap smear. She had always thought that regular Pap smears were unnecessary for women who were not sexually active. However, the magazine article she had read – written by a gynecologist – told her otherwise.

The gynecologist performs a pelvic examination and takes a cervical smear. Lisa is asked to call about the results the following week.

THE DIAGNOSIS
The laboratory reports abnormal cells in the smear, suggesting CARCINOMA IN SITU, a precancerous condition of the cervix. Although Lisa is worried, her gynecologist reassures her that this is only an early, mild form of cancer and that effective treatment is available.

THE TREATMENT
The gynecologist uses a colposcope (viewing instrument) to examine the surface of Lisa's cervix in detail. He finds a small area of abnormality and takes a sample (biopsy) to confirm that the cancer is in an early stage. A few days later, the diagnosis of carcinoma in situ is confirmed. Using a powerful laser beam, the doctor burns away the abnormal cells to expose the healthy tissue underneath. The treatment is painless.

THE OUTCOME
Although the carcinoma in situ has been removed, Lisa is asked to return in 1 month and then 3 months later for a pelvic examination and a Pap smear to ensure that the cancer hasn't returned. Thereafter, her doctor recommends that she have a Pap smear every 6 months.

Lisa is relieved that she went for the Pap test; if she had put it off, the cancer cells could have spread, making her condition more serious and the treatment not so simple.

Many women believe that they are at risk of cervical cancer only if they are sexually active. This is not true. Any woman – sexually active or not – is at risk and should have a Pap smear at regular intervals based on her doctor's recommendations. Cervical cancer is actually more common in older women.

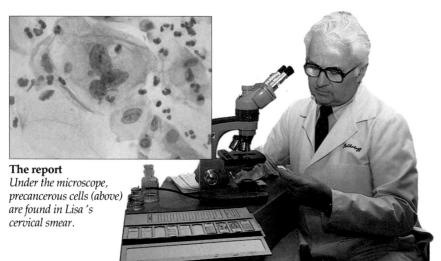

The report
Under the microscope, precancerous cells (above) are found in Lisa's cervical smear.

LUMBAR PUNCTURE

Although the advent of various scanning techniques has reduced the need for the lumbar puncture, it remains the standard method of obtaining a sample of cerebrospinal fluid, the watery fluid that bathes and cushions your brain and spinal cord. A cerebrospinal fluid sample is often vital in confirming a particular diagnosis because cerebrospinal fluid shows characteristic changes when specific diseases affecting the spinal cord or brain are present.

A rise in the pressure of the fluid can indicate the presence of a brain tumor, cerebral hemorrhage, acute meningitis, encephalitis, and other infections. Subarachnoid hemorrhage is a potentially dangerous condition in which blood leaks into the cerebrospinal fluid. Lumbar puncture can immediately reveal the presence of any blood. Also, normal cerebrospinal fluid contains few, if any, cells. If cells are detected during lumber puncture, their type and number can help confirm many disorders. In addition, the glucose and protein levels in the fluid have diagnostic value.

How is the sample taken?
You are asked to lie on your left side with your legs drawn up to your chest. Your doctor will ensure that your back is well curved. You should lie very still.

The skin of your back is swabbed with alcohol or an iodine solution, and sterile surgical drapes are placed around the site of the puncture. After an injection of a local anesthetic, a delicate, hollow needle, sealed with a metal stopper, is carefully inserted between two bones in the lumbar region of your spine until it enters the spinal canal. The doctor releases the stopper and attaches a glass tube attached to a pressure-measuring device so that the pressure of the fluid can be measured. He or she then allows a small quantity of cerebrospinal fluid to drip out into a sterile container.

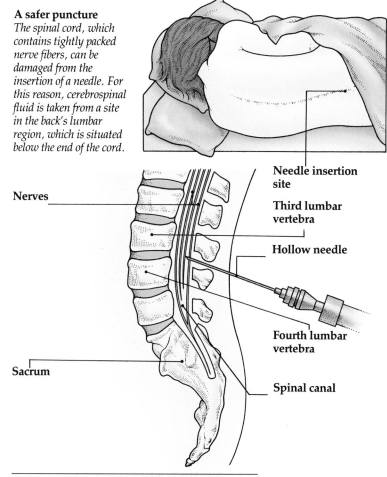

A safer puncture
The spinal cord, which contains tightly packed nerve fibers, can be damaged from the insertion of a needle. For this reason, cerebrospinal fluid is taken from a site in the back's lumbar region, which is situated below the end of the cord.

Nerves

Needle insertion site

Third lumbar vertebra

Hollow needle

Fourth lumbar vertebra

Sacrum

Spinal canal

JOINT ASPIRATION

If a joint has become swollen, aspiration is used to draw out a little of the synovial fluid that lubricates the joint, to help identify the cause of the swelling. The synovial fluid may be clear or opaque, watery or thick, and may contain blood or inflammatory cells and infectious organisms, which may be cultured.

How is the sample taken?
Joint aspiration is a simple procedure. The skin over your swollen joint is cleaned and drapes are applied. A local anesthetic is then injected into the joint. When the anesthetic has taken effect, a long needle, on another type of syringe, is passed carefully through the fibrous capsule that encloses the joint into the synovial fluid and a small quantity is drawn out. If the fluid is thick, the doctor may switch to a larger needle.

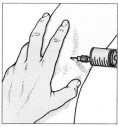

Aspiration
If gout is a suspected cause of arthritic pain, fluid may be aspirated from the joint for analysis.

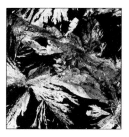

Excess uric acid
The microscope reveals crystals of uric acid, which causes gout.

BIOPSIES

Biopsies are samples of tissue that can be taken from any part of the body, even the brain. Laboratories usually require only a small sample of tissue for analysis. Brushing the area for a sample of cells (as is done in a Pap smear) is often sufficient. A needle and syringe are sometimes used, or a small area may be cut with a scalpel or by using the biopsy attachment of an endoscope. In other cases, a wide-diameter needle is used to take a core biopsy from a solid organ, such as the liver or kidney. A biopsy of the intestine may be taken by swallowing a capsule on the end of a line that is activated to cut a small slice when it reaches the correct section of intestine.

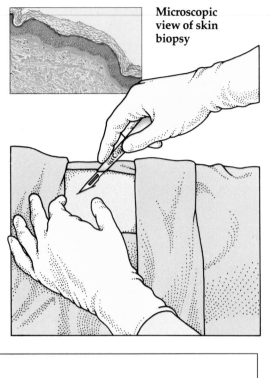

Microscopic view of skin biopsy

Skin biopsy
Investigation of irregularities of the skin may involve biopsy. A local anesthetic is given. Once it has taken effect a small part of the skin is cut out with a scalpel in such a way that the opening can be closed easily with a few stitches, leaving an almost invisible scar.

PROSTATE GLAND BIOPSY

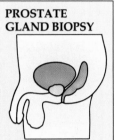

Prostate biopsy is done to confirm or exclude the diagnosis of prostatic cancer. It can be performed through the skin just in front of the anus, but the preferred route is through the wall of the rectum, from the inside, because the part of the gland adjacent to the rectum is the most prone to cancer.

You lie either on your side or on your back with your knees drawn up and your thighs wide apart. Your doctor uses a gloved finger to guide a special needle through your rectum into the prostate. The needle traps a tiny piece of the gland, which is withdrawn for analysis. Ultrasound imaging is sometimes used to help guide the needle to the area being biopsied.

PERFORMING A LIVER BIOPSY

A sample of liver tissue can confirm a diagnosis of cirrhosis, jaundice, chronic hepatitis, or a tumor or cyst in the liver.

For a liver biopsy, you are asked to lie along the edge of a bed with your right arm behind your head. You will be asked to stay in that position and remain as still as possible during the procedure. After the skin and the abdominal wall have been anesthetized, a needle is guided between two ribs as far as the liver surface. You are then asked to hold your breath and remain very still; a cough or sudden movement can cause the needle to tear your liver. Within seconds, the sample is taken.

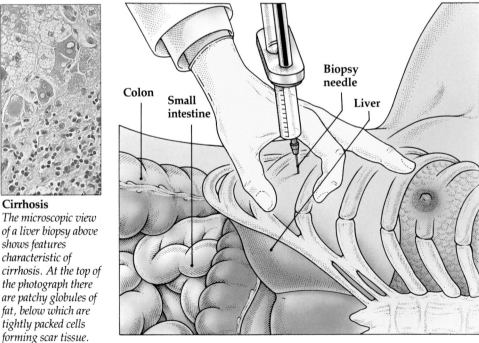

Cirrhosis
The microscopic view of a liver biopsy above shows features characteristic of cirrhosis. At the top of the photograph there are patchy globules of fat, below which are tightly packed cells forming scar tissue.

Colon   Small intestine   Biopsy needle   Liver

OBTAINING A BONE MARROW BIOPSY

A bone marrow biopsy is essential in the diagnosis of many blood, bone marrow, and lymphatic system disorders, including leukemias, tumors in the lymphatic system and bone marrow, unexplained anemias, and deficiencies of white blood cells.

Taking the biopsy
After you have been given a local anesthetic, a strong, short needle is guided through the skin and outer bone into the spongy center of the bone. A syringe is attached and a sample of the liquid bone marrow is drawn out (below). The sample is smeared onto glass slides and sent to the laboratory.

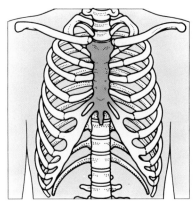

Biopsy sites
The biopsy is usually taken from the bone of the crest of the pelvis (below) or in some cases from your breastbone (above).

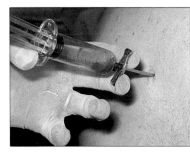

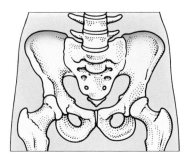

BREAST BIOPSY

If a mammogram or physical examination reveals a lump in the breast, the first step in deciding whether it is cancerous is usually a biopsy. The biopsy may be taken by inserting a needle into the lump; in some cases the entire lump is removed through a small, curved skin incision. For a larger lump, only a portion is taken. Fewer than one in five breast lumps is found to be cancerous.

Endometrial biopsy

This procedure is used to obtain tissue from the lining of the uterus. Examination of the sample supplies information about hormone balance. An endometrial biopsy can also locate a polyp or a malignant tumor, or any retained material from an early miscarriage.

The most common method, dilatation and curettage (D and C), is usually done with the use of a general anesthetic. A series of smooth, round-ended metal rods, of progressively increasing diameter, are used to widen the cervical canal of the uterus until the opening is wide enough to allow a curet – a small, sharp-edged spoon used to scrape away and remove some of the lining – to be passed into the uterus.

As an alternative, a delicate tube is passed through the cervical canal and a sample of uterine tissue is suctioned out. This method requires no anesthetic and can be done in the doctor's office.

ASK YOUR DOCTOR
TISSUE AND FLUID SAMPLES

Q **I recently had a biopsy of a mole on my back that my doctor was worried might be a malignant melanoma. The laboratory report said that my mole was not malignant – but how can I be sure that this is true?**

A For many conditions, the microscopic examination of a biopsy sample provides one of the most reliable methods of diagnosis. The person who examined your skin sample – a trained pathologist – is able to apply many sophisticated procedures, making the diagnosis almost certain.

Q **My father recently developed an abdominal swelling that his doctor says is due to fluid collection. He has been referred to the hospital to have some fluid drawn off it. How and why is this done?**

A The examination of fluid from the abdominal cavity (called peritoneal fluid analysis) can provide clues to possible heart, liver, or kidney disorders, as well as to the presence of tumors and infection of the peritoneum (lining of the cavity). The fluid is drawn off with the person lying down, rolled to one side to allow the fluid to gravitate. After an injection of a local anesthetic, a delicate needle or a syringe is used to withdraw the fluid. The procedure is painless.

Q **When do doctors recommend that a woman go to her doctor or clinic for her first Pap test?**

A The first test should be done before age 30 or soon after her first experience of sexual intercourse. Another test should be done 12 months later. Thereafter, Pap tests should be done every 3 years until the menopause and then every 3 to 5 years.

101

WHOLE BLOOD TESTS

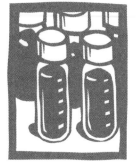

T HE BLOOD IS SO IMPORTANT to health that its study has become a complete specialty – hematology. A major portion of the work in a pathology laboratory concerns the range of different tests that can be performed on the blood. This section reviews the main tests performed on samples of whole blood.

Types of blood tests
When a blood sample arrives in the laboratory (below), tests may be carried out on whole blood (these tests are mainly concerned with the blood cells), on plasma (the part of whole blood that contains the dissolved clotting factors), or on serum (the straw-colored fluid that remains after whole blood has clotted).

Whole blood consists of a variety of cells suspended in a fluid called plasma. If a container of blood is allowed to clot, all the blood cells, and some of the proteins in the plasma, solidify, leaving a fluid known as serum. The specialty called serology focuses on measuring the substances present in serum (see CHEMICAL AND IMMUNOLOGICAL TESTS on page 108). Blood can also be cultured to detect and identify infectious organisms (see CULTURE AND MICROSCOPY on page 114).

Other tests performed on whole blood are primarily concerned with the quantity and quality of the blood cells and with the ability of the blood to clot.

BLOOD CELL TESTS

Red blood cells, called erythrocytes, are flat, concave-surfaced discs filled with the iron-containing protein hemoglobin, which carries oxygen in the blood. White blood cells play a major part in defending

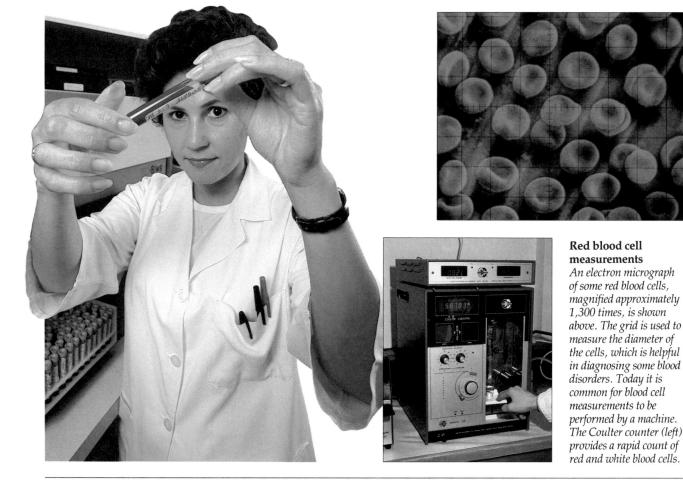

Red blood cell measurements
An electron micrograph of some red blood cells, magnified approximately 1,300 times, is shown above. The grid is used to measure the diameter of the cells, which is helpful in diagnosing some blood disorders. Today it is common for blood cell measurements to be performed by a machine. The Coulter counter (left) provides a rapid count of red and white blood cells.

the body against infection. Whole blood also contains numerous smaller cells, called platelets, that are important to blood clotting and the arrest of bleeding.

The doctor employs a range of tests to measure the quantity and quality of your blood cells. Today, many of these tests are performed automatically by a machine and a printout of the results is available in several minutes.

Red cell values

Two of the most important assessments made on the blood are the total red blood cell count – the number of red cells present in a cubic millimeter of blood – and the blood's hemoglobin concentration. The concentration of hemoglobin in the blood is reduced in all types of anemia, but the red cell count varies among the different types of anemia.

Hematocrit readings

If a sample of blood is put in a tube and spun rapidly in a centrifuge (a machine that uses the effect of centrifugal force), the red cells will pack together tightly and the percentage of the blood volume they take up – called the packed-cell volume or hematocrit – can be measured. Low hematocrit readings occur in most forms of anemia and (after a period of time) following severe bleeding. High readings occur in severe dehydration and after surgery, injury, and burns.

White blood cell count

The total number of white cells is counted and the relative number of different types of white cells (the white blood cell differential) may be measured.

The total white blood cell count increases with most bacterial infections and in certain other conditions, such as after bleeding and burns. A drop in the number of white cells follows certain types of poisoning, viral infections, and autoimmune diseases. Changes in the relative numbers of different types of white cells may indicate such diverse

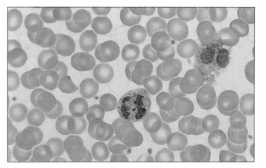

conditions as malaria and other parasitic diseases, viral infections, some types of cancer and leukemia, and allergies. The white cell count can also reveal to what stage the condition has progressed.

Blood smear

Examining the shape, size, and color of blood cells in a blood smear viewed under a microscope can provide an enormous amount of diagnostic information. Small, pale red cells suggest iron-deficiency anemia. Irregularities of red cell shape may suggest disorders such as pernicious anemia or sickle cell anemia. Abnormal-looking white cells can help diagnose various types of leukemia. These cells can also assist in the diagnosis of infectious mononucleosis.

Microscopic appearance of normal blood
If a drop of blood is allowed to fall onto a microscope slide and the edge of another slide is moved into the drop, the blood spreads along the edge and can then be drawn across the slide to form a thin film. This smear is stained first to bring out special features and is then examined under a microscope.

The blood smear shown here reveals many red cells (pale red discs), two stained white cells (with darker-stained nuclei), and a number of blood platelets (tiny purple particles). The cells are magnified about 800 times their actual size.

Sedimentation rate
The equipment at right is used to measure the rate at which blood is deposited as a sediment – an important measure called the erythrocyte (red blood cell) sedimentation rate (ESR).

Blood is drawn up into a calibrated tube, which is allowed to stand. After exactly 1 hour, the millimeters of clear serum above the red cell level represent the ESR.

The ESR is increased with certain infections, after a heart attack, with some kidney and thyroid diseases, and with many autoimmune diseases. It is not a highly specific test, but a high rate indicates that a disorder or disease is present.

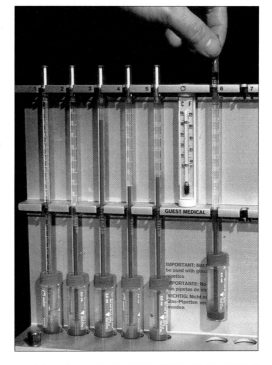

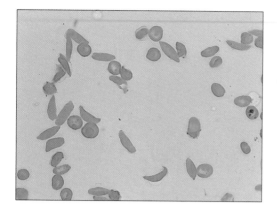

Microscopic examination
Many diseases that affect the blood can be diagnosed from abnormalities of the blood cells as seen under a microscope. Three examples are shown here.

Sickle cell anemia
In this condition, many red cells are deformed and have taken on elongated, sickle shapes. The disease is caused by an inherited abnormality of hemoglobin in the red blood cells.

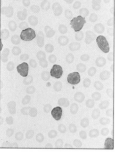

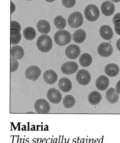

Acute lymphatic leukemia
In this type of cancer, there is an increased number of immature white cells (shown here stained purple) in the blood smear.

Malaria
This specially stained smear shows malaria parasites (pink areas) in virtually all the red blood cells (gray discs). The parasites are transmitted by mosquito bites.

Examining a specially stained blood smear may also reveal bacteria (in septicemia or blood poisoning) and the parasites responsible for such tropical diseases as malaria and sleeping sickness.

Complete blood count

A complete blood count is a compilation of several of the tests mentioned on page 103 plus the platelet count. The overall blood picture may give a more reliable diagnosis than is possible from the results of one or two tests alone.

BLOOD CLOTTING TESTS

When a blood vessel is injured, a clot normally forms at the site of injury. The principal components of the blood clotting system are the platelet particles, and the clotting factors, which are proteins in the blood plasma. Deficiency or malfunc-

tion of either of these blood components can cause a tendency to bleed.

When investigating bleeding disorders, a complete blood count, including a platelet count, is done first. It may reveal a low platelet count as an isolated finding or as one of several different abnormalities.

Specific tests

After a complete blood count, a variety of tests may be performed to evaluate the severity of the clotting abnormality and to identify possible deficiencies of clotting factors in the blood. The tests may reveal an inherited deficiency of a particular clotting factor (as occurs in hemophilia, caused by deficiency of clotting factor VIII) or may indicate a disorder of the liver, which produces many of the clotting factors.

More sophisticated measures to evaluate clotting involve adding different anti-clotting and pro-clotting substances to blood samples and then timing how long the samples take to clot. By comparing the results of two or more tests, the number of possible causes of a bleeding disorder can be narrowed.

CASE HISTORY
FATIGUE AND WEIGHT LOSS

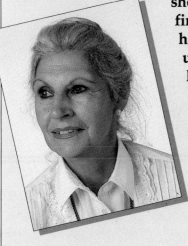

FOR THE LAST SEVERAL MONTHS, **Paula has been losing weight and has become increasingly tired and breathless after only minor exertion. She also thinks that she is losing the sensation in her fingers and her toes. Her husband has noticed that she has become unusually pale and that her skin has a distinct lemon yellow color. Eventually he persuades her to see a doctor.**

PERSONAL DETAILS
Name Paula Anderson
Age 63
Occupation Lawyer
Family No history of significant disease.

MEDICAL BACKGROUND
Paula had breast cancer at age 47 and had a radical mastectomy; there has been no recurrence.

THE CONSULTATION
Paula tells the doctor that she has become so weak that she staggers when she walks. Her tongue is sore, her fingers tingle, and she is anxious because she can't concentrate on her court cases.

The doctor notes her obvious loss of weight and yellow skin color, and checks the insides of her lower eyelids, which are very pale. She tests Paula's muscle strength and finds that she is much weaker than normal. The doctor then checks her sensitivity to touch and finds it is almost absent in her legs and hands.

FURTHER INVESTIGATION
A blood sample is taken for blood cell tests and measurement of vitamin B_{12}. The doctor also takes a sample of fluid from Paula's stomach and sends it for analysis.

The results of the tests are revealing. Paula's gastric juice contains no acid. The blood test shows that many of her red cells are much larger than normal and that some of them have an irregular shape. Paula's total red cell count is severely reduced and the amount of vitamin B_{12} in her blood is extremely low.

THE DIAGNOSIS
A bone marrow biopsy confirms the doctor's suspicion that Paula is suffering from PERNICIOUS ANEMIA. This type of anemia is caused by an inability of the intestines to absorb vitamin B_{12} from food. And because vitamin B_{12} is essential for the production of red blood cells, Paula's bone marrow is failing to produce red cells normally.

A degenerative condition of the nervous system has also developed as a result of the vitamin B_{12} deficiency. This accounts for the tingling, loss of sensation, weakness, and occasional mental confusion.

THE TREATMENT
Paula is given hydroxycobalamin, a form of vitamin B_{12}. She takes it daily for a week, weekly for 3 months, and then monthly.

THE OUTCOME
In less than 3 months Paula's red cell count has been restored to a normal level, and signs of anemia such as her pallor and sore tongue have disappeared. Paula feels more energetic than she has in years and, although full sensation has not returned to her legs, her muscle strength has improved. Best of all, she is now as alert as ever and won her last court case.

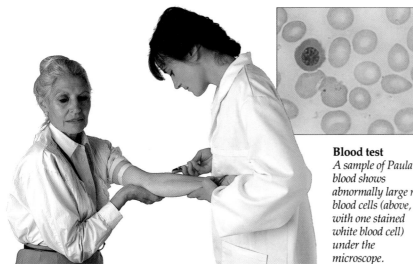

Blood test
A sample of Paula's blood shows abnormally large red blood cells (above, with one stained white blood cell) under the microscope.

WHAT'S IN A DROP OF BLOOD?

For diagnosing disease, your blood is by far the most important body fluid. Each drop of blood is a veritable "soup" containing hundreds of different constituents – cells, proteins, and individual chemicals – all suspended or dissolved in water. Different diseases cause alterations in the levels or appearance of these constituents, which can provide vital clues to diagnosis.

The only normal constituents of blood visible under a light microscope are the blood cells and platelets, shown here at up to 10,000 times actual size. Proteins and individual chemicals (far right) have molecules that are about 500 to 50,000 times smaller than blood cells, so they can be detected and measured only by chemical tests.

White blood cells

White blood cells, which take several different forms, are key components of the body's immune system; they function to defend the body against infection. Some of them directly attack and engulf invading microbes, while others produce antibodies that attack the microbes. The appearance of the white cells under a microscope, and a count of their relative numbers, can assist in the diagnosis of leukemia, many infectious diseases, and immune system disorders.

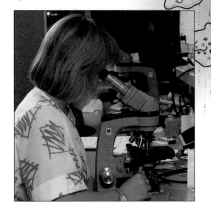

Light microscope
Red and white blood cells can be clearly seen at a magnification of about 200.

Red blood cells
These disc-shaped cells are packed with the oxygen-carrying substance hemoglobin, which gives blood its red color. The appearance of red cells under a microscope, and laboratory measurements of their hemoglobin content and numbers in the blood, can aid in the diagnosis of various forms of anemia.

Platelets
When a blood vessel wall is injured, these tiny particles aid in the arrest of bleeding by sticking to each other and plugging the break in the vessel wall. In the laboratory, the number of platelets in the blood (and their "stickiness") is measured to help in the diagnosis of disorders that cause abnormal bleeding.

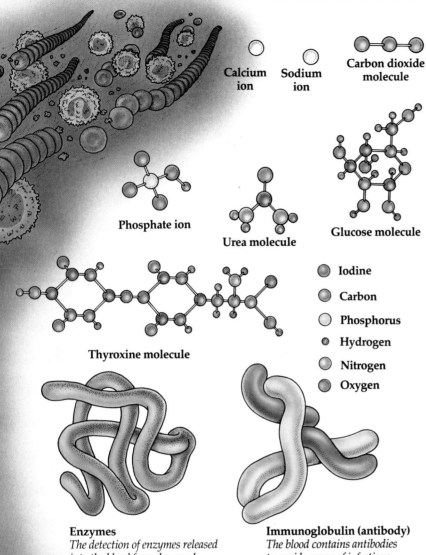

Calcium ion

Sodium ion

Carbon dioxide molecule

Phosphate ion

Urea molecule

Glucose molecule

- Iodine
- Carbon
- Phosphorus
- Hydrogen
- Nitrogen
- Oxygen

Thyroxine molecule

Enzymes
The detection of enzymes released into the blood from damaged tissues can aid in the diagnosis of heart, liver, muscle, pancreatic, and prostatic disorders. The shape of a typical enzyme molecule is shown above.

Immunoglobulin (antibody)
The blood contains antibodies to a wide range of infections. Measuring the level of antibodies in the blood can aid in the diagnosis of infectious diseases and immune system disorders.

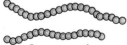
Streptococci

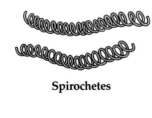
Spirochetes

Bacteria and viruses
Bacteria, such as streptococci or spirochetes, can sometimes be seen in the blood under a microscope; their presence may also be confirmed by laboratory culture of a sample of blood. Viruses (right) can be seen in the blood only with an electron microscope – but viral infection can often be confirmed by chemical detection of antibodies formed against the viruses.

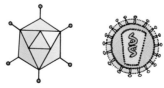
Hepatitis virus   **HIV (AIDS virus)**

Measuring Chemicals

Individual chemicals with small to medium-sized molecules in the blood include gases such as carbon dioxide; nutrients such as glucose, amino acids, and cholesterol; hormones such as thyroxine; waste products such as urea; and ions such as sodium, calcium, and phosphate. Measuring the individual substances by chemical means can help in the diagnosis of endocrine (glandular) disorders and kidney, liver, and lung disease.

Counting Proteins

Proteins are large, complex molecules. Many types are present in blood, including albumin (which helps maintain blood volume), immunoglobulins (antibodies), clotting factors, enzymes (catalytic proteins), and some hormones such as insulin. Abnormal levels of specific proteins in the blood can aid in the diagnosis of a vast range of disorders, including some cancers and diseases of the liver and kidneys.

Detecting Invaders

Microbes such as bacteria, viruses, and protozoa (single-celled parasites) are not normally present in blood. However, in certain infections, their presence can be detected to help clinch a diagnosis.

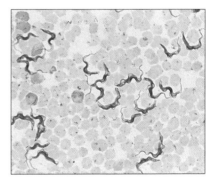

Parasites
In diseases such as malaria and sleeping sickness, the causative parasites can sometimes be seen in the blood under a light microscope. Shown above are some purple-stained trypanosomes (the cause of sleeping sickness) in a blood smear.

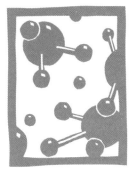

CHEMICAL AND IMMUNOLOGICAL TESTS

C HEMICAL AND IMMUNOLOGICAL TESTS on blood and other body fluids can provide important clues to the diagnosis of a wide range of diseases, including disorders of major body organs, such as the heart, liver, and kidneys, hormonal disorders, infectious diseases, and disorders of the immune system.

Because so many different chemical tests are performed in laboratories today, only a selection can be discussed here. Many more tests are described briefly in the A–Z OF MEDICAL TESTS on pages 128 to 141.

CHEMICAL TESTS

Blood is the most important body fluid in terms of the number of tests performed on it and the amount of information that can be gathered from it. Many of the substances in blood are filtered into the urine, making tests on urine samples significant as well.

Blood gases

The function of the lungs is to take oxygen from inhaled air and bring it into close contact with the blood, where red blood cells take up the oxygen. The blood also carries carbon dioxide, one of the body's main waste products, from the tissues back to the lungs so that it can be breathed out. This makes the state of the gases (oxygen and carbon dioxide) in your blood an important factor.

The amount of oxygen and carbon dioxide in the blood is usually measured in a fresh sample of blood obtained from an artery. In conditions of respiratory

In the laboratory
Individual chemical and immunological testing of samples by hand has become uncommon in an age of automation. Instead, most chemical analyses today are performed by machine. Here a technician loads samples into a machine that measures tiny amounts of hormones in the blood and urine.

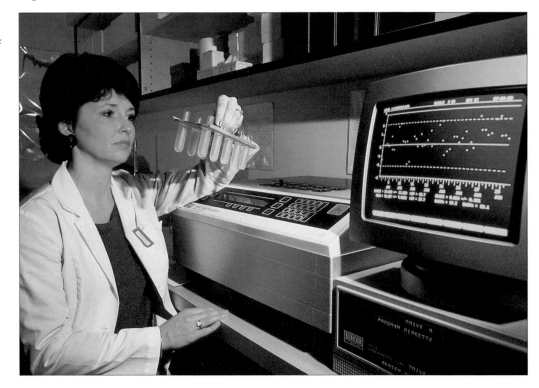

distress, such as emphysema or an asthma attack, and in some forms of congenital heart disease, the blood oxygen level is low and the carbon dioxide level is high. Blood gas evaluation is fundamental to the management of many heart and lung disorders.

Blood electrolytes

The blood contains many simple compounds that break down in solution to form electrically charged particles called ions. A substance such as sodium chloride (table salt) breaks down into positively charged sodium ions (Na+) and negatively charged chloride ions (Cl-). Because these ions can be caused to move by the application of an electric current, they are called electrolytes.

Electrolytes such as calcium, sodium, potassium, phosphate, and chloride must be present in the correct concentrations if the body is to function properly; the body's regulating mechanisms ensure that, in a healthy person, they do so. Many diseases, such as some kidney and endocrine (hormonal) gland disorders, result in a change in the electrolyte levels, so measuring the levels of electrolytes in the blood and sometimes in the urine can be informative.

Albumin

Albumin is an important protein in blood that helps maintain blood volume and prevents water from accumulating in tissues. Its level is diminished in liver disease and in some kidney disease. The presence of albumin and other proteins in the urine indicates kidney damage.

Blood enzymes

Enzymes are proteins that cause chemical reactions to accelerate; they are essential for the normal functioning of the body. When body cells are damaged, some enzymes escape into the blood, where their concentration can be measured. This can provide valuable information about the presence and degree of

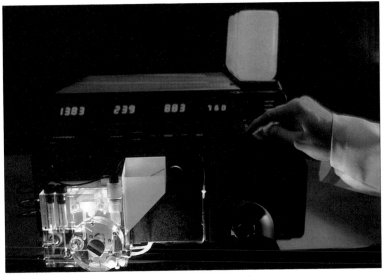

damage to organs such as the heart and liver. Some of the important enzymes, along with their associated disorders, are listed in the table below.

Nutrients

One of the most important nutrients in the blood is glucose. Excess glucose in the blood and urine usually indicates diabetes mellitus, in which the pancreas produces either an insufficient amount of the hormone insulin or, in insulin-dependent people, no insulin at all. Insulin is vital to the body's use of glucose.

Blood gas and pH analyzer
The analyzer shown above is specifically designed to measure gases (oxygen and carbon dioxide) in blood samples and the blood's acid-base balance (pH). Some laboratories use larger machines that are able to process hundreds of blood samples simultaneously.

IMPORTANT BLOOD ENZYMES	
ENZYME	DISORDERS INCREASING LEVELS
Alanine aminotransferase (ALT)	Heart, liver, or muscle damage
Aspartate aminotransferase (AST)	Liver, heart, or muscle damage
Gamma-glutamyl transferase (GGT)	Liver damage and, in some cases, pancreatic disease
Alkaline phosphatase	Liver damage, bone disease, and overactivity of the parathyroid glands
Acid phosphatase	Cancer of the prostate gland
Amylase	Inflammation of the pancreas
Lactate dehydrogenase	Myocardial infarction (heart attack) or some types of cancer, anemia, and muscle and kidney disease
Creatine kinase (CK)	Muscle damage or degeneration

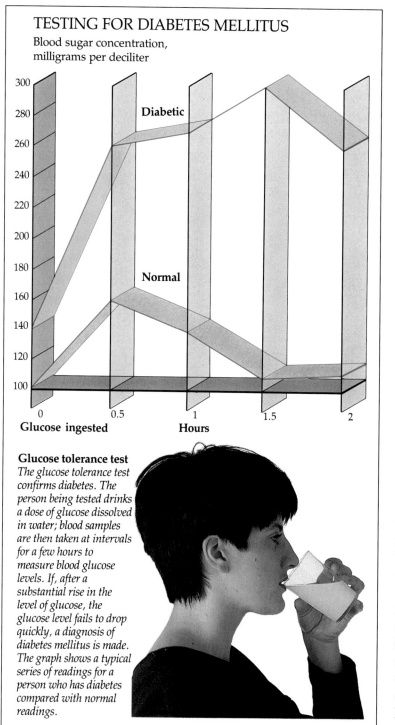

TESTING FOR DIABETES MELLITUS

Blood sugar concentration, milligrams per deciliter

Diabetic

Normal

0   0.5   1   1.5   2

Glucose ingested   **Hours**

Glucose tolerance test
The glucose tolerance test confirms diabetes. The person being tested drinks a dose of glucose dissolved in water; blood samples are then taken at intervals for a few hours to measure blood glucose levels. If, after a substantial rise in the level of glucose, the glucose level fails to drop quickly, a diagnosis of diabetes mellitus is made. The graph shows a typical series of readings for a person who has diabetes compared with normal readings.

Hormones

Measuring hormones in the blood and urine can be important in the diagnosis of disorders caused by underactivity or overactivity of the body's endocrine glands. The activity of several glands, notably the thyroid gland, adrenal glands, ovaries, and testes, is controlled by the secretion of hormones from the pituitary gland – the master gland in the brain. When a doctor is investigating thyroid disease, he or she may request that a battery of tests (called thyroid function tests) be performed. These tests can measure the controlling hormone secreted by the pituitary (thyroid-stimulating hormone) as well as hormones secreted by the thyroid itself (thyroxine and triiodothyronine). Similar blood and urine tests – adrenal function tests, pituitary function tests, or gonadal function tests – are used to investigate other glandular disorders.

Liver and kidney function tests

When liver or kidney disease is suspected, a variety of chemical tests may be performed to evaluate the function of these organs. Tests for the liver include those for certain enzymes, and for bilirubin and albumin in the blood, and blood clotting tests (the liver manufactures blood clotting factors).

Bilirubin is a pigment released when red blood cells are broken down either at the end of their normal life span or earlier in some disease processes. Bilirubin is normally processed in the liver and excreted in the bile. However, if the liver is diseased or the outflow of bile from the liver is blocked, bilirubin is returned to the blood. Thus, measuring the level of bilirubin in the blood can give an indication of the severity of liver damage or bile duct obstruction.

Kidney function tests include measurements of the waste products urea and creatinine in the blood and urine to determine whether these substances are being efficiently filtered from the blood.

Other nutrients that may be measured in the blood include amino acids (raised levels may indicate liver or kidney disease or certain genetic disorders), vitamins (reduced levels may indicate vitamin deficiency disease), and cholesterol (a raised level may signify an increased risk of artery and heart disease).

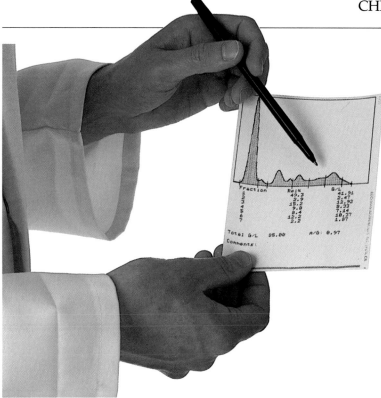

Urea is one of the primary breakdown products of protein; it moves from the blood to the kidneys, where it is excreted in the urine. A rise in the urea level indicates malfunctioning of the kidneys.

In addition, urine may be examined for blood cells, pus cells, protein, and casts (cells and mucuslike material shed from damaged kidney tissue). The presence of any of these cells or materials in the urine may indicate kidney disease.

Fecal tests

One of the most important chemical tests done on feces is the fecal occult blood test. This test checks for hidden traces of blood in the feces. Traces of blood may occur in diseases such as peptic ulcer, dysentery, or cancer of the stomach or colon. The test is performed by applying a paper strip or tablet to a fecal sample. Certain foods (such as red meat) and supplements (such as vitamin C) must be avoided before the test because they can cause false results. The fat content of feces is also tested and can be helpful in diagnosing disorders in which fats are poorly absorbed from the intestines, which results in persistent diarrhea.

Blood protein analysis
The doctor is holding a chart that gives a breakdown of proteins in the blood, obtained by a technique called electrophoresis. This technique uses an electric field to separate different proteins on a sheet of paper. Proteins in the blood include albumin, immunoglobulins (antibodies), enzymes, and some hormones. Measuring them can give clues to liver, kidney, and immune system disease.

IMMUNOLOGICAL TESTS

Immunology is the branch of medicine concerned with the immune system – the body's defenses against infection. When infectious agents enter the body, proteins on their surfaces (called antigens) are recognized as foreign by the immune system, which provokes certain white blood cells to produce substances called antibodies or immunoglobulins.

These bind on to and inactivate the antigens, destroying them. Other white cells directly attack the invaders.

Immunological tests are concerned with antibody/antigen reactions and are used in the diagnosis of three broad categories of disease – infectious diseases, allergies, and autoimmune diseases.

Testing for infections

Many infectious diseases are diagnosed by looking for infectious organisms

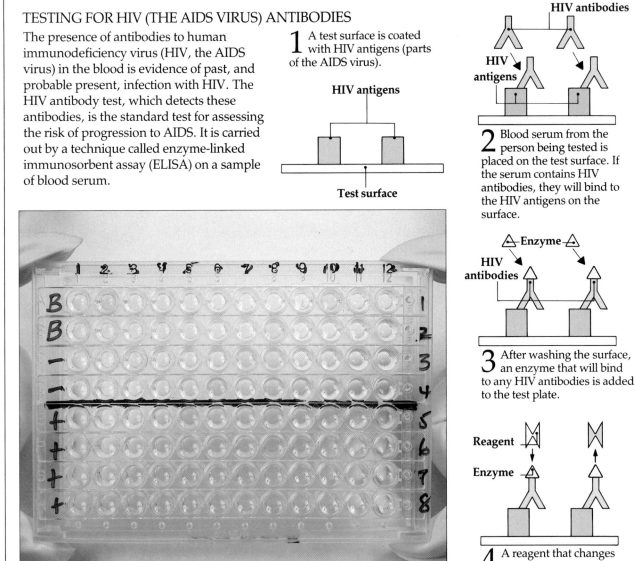

TESTING FOR HIV (THE AIDS VIRUS) ANTIBODIES

The presence of antibodies to human immunodeficiency virus (HIV, the AIDS virus) in the blood is evidence of past, and probable present, infection with HIV. The HIV antibody test, which detects these antibodies, is the standard test for assessing the risk of progression to AIDS. It is carried out by a technique called enzyme-linked immunosorbent assay (ELISA) on a sample of blood serum.

1 A test surface is coated with HIV antigens (parts of the AIDS virus).

HIV antigens

Test surface

2 Blood serum from the person being tested is placed on the test surface. If the serum contains HIV antibodies, they will bind to the HIV antigens on the surface.

HIV antibodies

HIV antigens

3 After washing the surface, an enzyme that will bind to any HIV antibodies is added to the test plate.

Enzyme

HIV antibodies

4 A reagent that changes color when it comes in contact with the enzyme is added. Color change indicates that the enzyme (and therefore HIV antibodies) is present.

Reagent

Enzyme

Test plate
The test plate above consists of several wells, each of which has a surface that can be used for an individual HIV antibody test. Samples of blood serum from different people are added to the wells, giving positive (yellow) and negative (clear) results for the presence of HIV antibodies.

IMMUNOASSAYS

Immunoassays are a group of sensitive measuring techniques. Just as the body's immune system produces antibodies that bind to specific proteins (antigens) in the blood, so known antibodies (or antigens) can be used to detect antigens or antibodies in blood samples, provided the binding of antibodies and antigens can be measured in the laboratory.

In radioimmuno-assay (RIA), a radioactively labeled substance that will attach to antibody/antigen complexes is employed. Enzyme-linked immunosorbent assay (ELISA) is a related type of immunoassay used for the HIV antibody test (see box at left).

under a microscope or by culturing the organisms (see CULTURE AND MICROSCOPY on page 114). However, other infections, particularly those caused by small organisms such as viruses or rickettsiae, are more easily confirmed by testing for a rising level of antibodies in the blood. All of us have low levels of antibodies to many different organisms, but this does not necessarily indicate a recent or current infection. However, if your doctor takes a blood sample early in the course of a disease and then another about 2 or 3 weeks later, and a difference is found in the levels of the two samples, an infection is indicated.

Important viral diseases that can be confirmed by immunological testing include viral hepatitis, viral meningitis, herpes infections, and HIV (the AIDS virus) infection. Rickettsial diseases include Rocky Mountain spotted fever, typhus, and Q fever.

Testing for allergies

Allergies are caused by inappropriate reactions of the immune system to certain innocuous substances (allergens) that enter the body. The immune system produces antibodies to these allergens as though they were foreign antigens. Skin tests are usually the first tests for allergies. They are highly reliable for most people. When skin tests cannot be used, the radioallergosorbent test, which specifically detects the presence of antibodies to allergens, may be employed. In this test the person's blood serum is brought into contact with known allergens on a series of test plates. The formation of antibody/allergen complexes is detected by adding a radioactively labeled substance that binds to the complexes on the test plates.

Testing for autoimmune disease

In autoimmune diseases, such as rheumatoid arthritis, systemic lupus erythematosus, some types of thyroid disease, and pernicious anemia, the immune system produces antibodies that attack the body's tissues, interfering with their function and destroying them. Diagnosing these disorders may be assisted by testing the blood for the relevant antibodies. In rheumatoid arthritis, the blood is tested for a group of antibodies called rheumatoid factor.

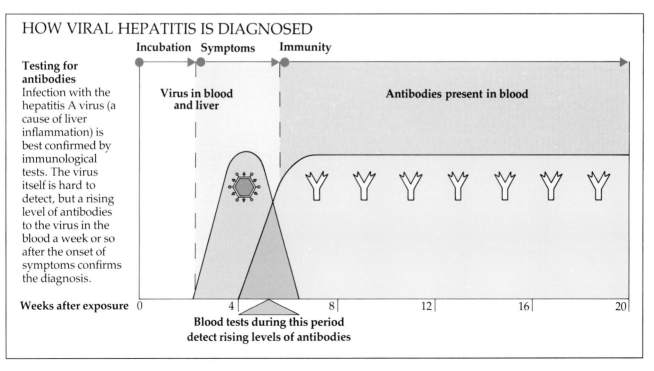

HOW VIRAL HEPATITIS IS DIAGNOSED

Testing for antibodies
Infection with the hepatitis A virus (a cause of liver inflammation) is best confirmed by immunological tests. The virus itself is hard to detect, but a rising level of antibodies to the virus in the blood a week or so after the onset of symptoms confirms the diagnosis.

Incubation Symptoms Immunity

Virus in blood and liver

Antibodies present in blood

Weeks after exposure 0 4 8 12 16 20

Blood tests during this period detect rising levels of antibodies

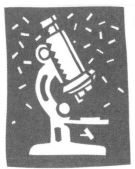

CULTURE AND MICROSCOPY

T O HELP ESTABLISH the cause of an infection, samples of fluid or tissue are cultured in the laboratory to grow, test for, and identify bacteria and fungi. Samples are also examined under the microscope for a variety of microorganisms, and tissue obtained by biopsy is examined for evidence of disease.

Microorganisms that cause disease in the human body fall into several groups. The most important are bacteria, viruses, and fungi; three smaller groups, the rickettsiae, chlamydiae, and mycoplasmas, are also important. Other groups include the protozoa (single-celled animal parasites) and the eggs and larvae of a variety of parasitic worms. Disease-causing microorganisms are called pathogens.

Culture is the standard method of producing an uncontaminated sample of bacteria for identification. To a lesser extent, fungi are also cultured to produce a pure specimen whenever a fungal infection is suspected. Cultures for many viruses and chlamydiae can also be performed, though they entail more complicated laboratory procedures. Certain viruses and rickettsiae are difficult to cul-

Examining bacteria
When giving a sample for culture, your doctor tells the microbiologist the type of bacterial infection suspected. An agar medium for the suspected organism is selected and inoculated and, after about a day, colonies of bacteria may be visible.

Growing the bacteria
The agar plate at left shows a colony of streptococci bacteria. Salmonella bacteria are growing on the plate shown below. Bacteria from a single colony are transferred to a fresh agar plate so that a pure amount of the bacteria can be grown and used for specific identification testing and antibiotic susceptibility testing.

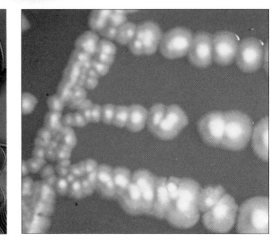

ture, so, whenever one of these microorganisms is suspected of causing disease, the serum of the patient is tested for the development of antibodies to the suspected microorganism. Protozoa, worms, eggs, and larvae are usually readily visible under the microscope; the trained observer can immediately recognize them without testing further.

CULTURING BACTERIA

Your skin, intestines, throat, and genitals are swarming with bacteria. Most of these bacteria are not only harmless, they help keep dangerous, disease-causing bacteria at bay. It is one of the tasks of a bacteriologist to distinguish pathogenic bacteria from the harmless bacteria and other safe microorganisms that may be found in a specimen.

If you have an infection and your doctor suspects that your infection has a bacterial cause, he or she may take a sample from the site of infection, such as a fecal sample if the colon is infected or a swab from the surface of the eye if the conjunctiva is infected. The sample is then sent with any diagnostic information to the microbiology laboratory for a confirmatory culture. Samples of blood, urine, sputum, and vaginal or urethral discharges, and swabs from wounds, the throat, and other areas, such as the mouth, skin, and outer-ear canal, can also be sent for culture.

How are bacteria cultured?

In the laboratory, a swab from the sample is smeared across the surface of a special gel contained in a shallow, covered, glass dish. The culture gel is the seaweed-based agar; bacteria grow well on the agar surface. Agar is used because, much like gelatin, it liquefies when heated (during sterilization) and solidifies again at room temperature. A blood or meat extract is often added to the heated mix to produce a more nutritious medium for the growth of bacteria.

THE ANTIBIOTIC SENSITIVITY TEST

The bacteria are resistant to these antibiotics

The bacteria are not resistant (are "sensitive") to these antibiotics

Once colonies of bacteria have formed in a glass dish, the bacteriologist can create pure subcultures by transferring colonies via a sterile wire loop to another agar dish. It is then possible not only to identify the organisms but to perform tests on the pure colonies to determine their resistance (sensitivity) to various antibiotics. An agar plate is heavily smeared with a pure culture of bacteria and then a set of small paper discs, each impregnated with a different antibiotic, is dropped onto the culture plate. After a while there are clear zones, free of bacterial growth, around those antibiotics that kill the organisms; bacteria are not resistant to these antibiotics. This procedure, called the antibiotic sensitivity test, is a great help to the doctor in deciding the best antibiotic to treat your condition.

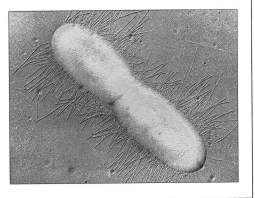

Escherichia coli
The bacteria growing in the culture above belong to the species Escherichia coli, *one cause of urinary tract infection. A single dividing bacterium, magnified approximately 15,000 times, is shown in the color-enhanced electron micrograph at right.*

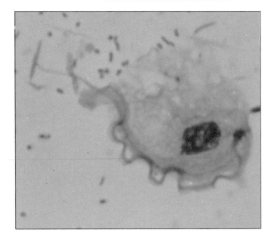

Trichomonas vaginalis
Visible in this urine sample is the single-cell protozoon microbe Trichomonas vaginalis, *which commonly infects the mucous membrane of the vagina, causing irritation and discharge. The microbe was easily transported from the vaginal area into the urine during urination.*

Urethritis
The bacteria in this urine sample are of the species Proteus mirabilis, *a common cause of inflammation of the urethra. Unlike many bacteria, the species has delicate hairs that help it move and spread around the area of infection.*

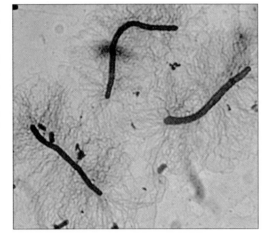

If the doctor suspects a particular organism, a special culture medium with specific additives may be chosen to encourage the growth of that organism and discourage the growth of others. The agar dish is then put into an incubator kept at 37°C (body temperature) because organisms pathogenic to humans grow best at this temperature. The culture may show a mixed growth of bacterial colonies, but those of the bacterial infection usually predominate over those colonies that are harmless and nonpathogenic.

BACTERIOLOGICAL MICROSCOPY

Bacteria can be taken from a pure culture, or even taken directly from your body fluid, secretions, or tissue sample, and spread on a slide, dried, and then stained for examination.

One universally used stain, Gram's stain, can divide all bacteria into two large groups. The gram-positive organisms are those that stain dark purple; gram-negative organisms stain red. The gram-positive group includes the staphylococci, which cause boils, toxic shock syndrome, pneumonia, and wound infection; the streptococci, which

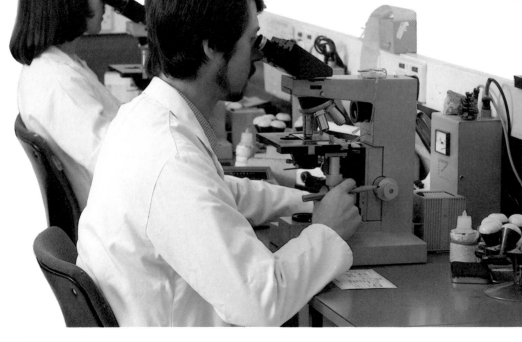

Examining pathogens
The trained observer, who has viewed thousands of samples of body fluids and tissues under the microscope, is familiar with the characteristics of a wide variety of disease-causing microorganisms. The instrument being used here is a standard light microscope, which provides a magnification of up to 1,500 times. The glass slide containing the specimen is placed on a platform called a stage, and an optical condenser situated underneath the stage concentrates light from a built-in illuminator upward onto the specimen.

cause sore throat, blood infection, and inflammation of the lining of the heart; the anthrax bacillus; and the clostridia, which cause tetanus and gas gangrene.

The gram-negative group includes many of the bacteria that infect the bowel, such as the salmonellae, shigellae, and *Campylobacter* organisms; *Legionella pneumophilia*, which causes legionnaires' disease; the *Meningococcus* bacterium, which causes meningitis; the whooping cough bacterium; and the gonococci, which cause gonorrhea. Many gram-negative organisms also can cause urinary tract infections and blood infections in chronically ill people.

Other identification tests

It is sometimes necessary to perform more tests to identify bacteria. For example, the normal bacteria of the bowel and the various bacteria that cause diarrhea and dysentery are all gram-negative and look alike under the microscope. However, each of these organisms is able to ferment a different set of sugar nutrients. Again, a pure culture of an organism is put into tubes of several different sugars and the pattern of sugar fermentation identifies the bacterial species accurately. For example, the bacterium *Escherichia coli* ferments lactose, but the salmonellae and the shigellae dysentery organisms do not.

MICROSCOPY FOR FUNGI, PROTOZOA, AND WORMS

Microorganisms that are roughly the same size, or larger, than bacteria can also be identified under a microscope. As with bacteria, various stains can be used to help reveal the organisms. Fungi such as *Candida albicans* (the cause of thrush) can be identified by microscopy from oral and genital swabs. The protozoa responsible for malaria, amebic dysentery (an infection of the intestines), and trichomoniasis (a sexually transmitted disease that causes a vaginal discharge)

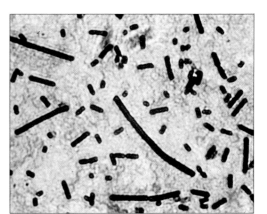

Typhoid
This specimen of diarrheal fluid contains the bacilli (rod-shaped bacteria) of Salmonella typhosa, *the cause of typhoid fever. Other bacteria of the same genus are responsible for paratyphoid fever and different types of food poisoning.*

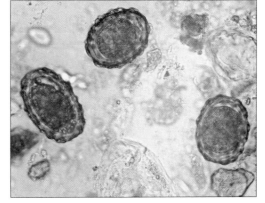

Roundworm
This fecal sample contains eggs of the roundworm Ascaris lumbricoides, *a parasite of the human intestine found in many parts of the world. The worm is usually acquired by swallowing food or licking fingers that have been contaminated by the roundworm eggs.*

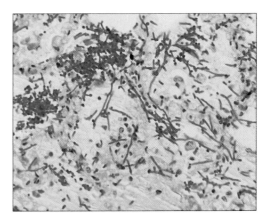

Thrush
In this color-enhanced slide of tissue taken from the tongue, there are long threads of the fungus Candida albicans, *the cause of thrush. The fungus infects the mucous membranes of the mouth and vagina, causing a thick, white coating to form.*

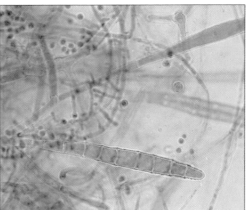

Athletes' foot
In this tissue sample taken from between the fourth and fifth toes, the microscope reveals a fungus of the Trichophyton *genus, which causes the fungal infection athletes' foot. The fungus is spread in warm, moist, communal areas where clothes are changed.*

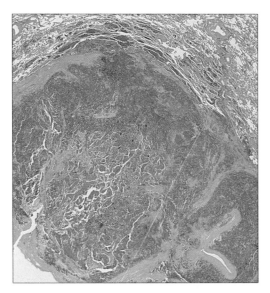

Lung tumor
In this color-enhanced light micrograph, an oat-cell carcinoma (the blue-stained material) is growing into and destroying a bronchus (airway) of the lung. It is called an oat-cell carcinoma because the tightly packed, oval cells of the tumor resemble oat seeds when viewed at high magnification.

Emphysema
This slide shows lung tissue from a person with emphysema. The light areas are air spaces. They are larger than those of normal lung tissue because the disease has caused the membranes between them to break down. In the center of the slide, a section of a vein containing blood is visible.

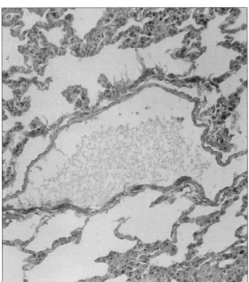

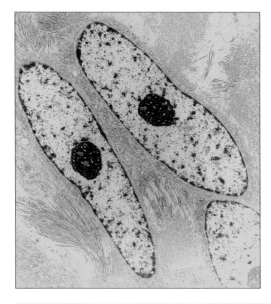

Spindle-cell sarcoma
In this color-enhanced slide, two spindle cells from a human sarcoma (cancerous tumor) are shown. The dark-stained circular areas are the large nuclei. Unlike many other cancer cells, these malignant spindle cells have little similarity to the tissue cells from which they originated.

can be identified from blood, fecal samples, and genital secretions, respectively. Eggs of the common roundworm, hookworms, and other worms that parasitize the intestines can be identified from fecal samples; eggs of the fluke responsible for the tropical disease schistosomiasis (bilharziasis) can be seen in a sample of the infested person's urine.

Microorganisms that are much smaller than bacteria – viruses, chlamydiae, and rickettsiae – are too small to be seen with a standard microscope. Although some organisms can be identified with an electron microscope, infections with these organisms are usually identified by culture tests and by testing the affected person's blood serum to look for antibodies that the immune system has produced to attack these organisms (see IMMUNOLOGICAL TESTS on page 112).

CELL AND TISSUE EXAMINATION

The microscope is not used solely to detect and identify pathogenic microorganisms. In fact, its principal use for diagnostic purposes is to study the cellular structure and function of abnormal body tissues (histopathology) and of abnormal individual body cells (cytopathology).

Diagnosing disease from the appearance of tissue and cell preparations under the microscope is usually clearcut. For example, an experienced pathologist can identify a malignant tumor at a glance from a tissue slice. Cancer cells typically have large nuclei and form irregular patterns, distorting blood vessels and other healthy structures.

How is tissue prepared?
Tissue obtained by biopsy is first examined by a pathologist, who submits the appropriate portions, which are then fixed in formalin or similar fixatives, for diagnosis. The fixed tissue is then soaked in melted paraffin wax and allowed to cool and harden into a block. A

precision instrument called a microtome is used to cut wafer-thin slices from the block; these slices are then mounted on glass slides. The wax is dissolved out of the tissue with a solvent, and the specimen is stained to enhance the microscopic detail. A pathologist then examines the slide under a microscope and writes a report on the findings.

To examine individual cells such as those taken in a Pap smear, the sample or swab is smeared onto the slide, fixed, stained with dyes to show cell details, and then examined under the microscope by a cytotechnologist or physician cytopathologist.

How long does it take?

A biopsy result may take from a few days to a week to prepare and interpret, especially if additional tissue sections or special staining procedures are required for accurate diagnosis.

In cases of extreme urgency, usually during an operation, a report may be obtained within half an hour by freezing the tissue and cutting slices from the frozen block, while the patient remains anesthetized on the operating table. In these cases, the surgeon's actions depend on what the pathologist finds.

Leukemia
This microscope photograph of a bone marrow smear shows evidence of leukemia, a malignant disease of the white blood cells. The cells stained purple are immature forms of one type of white blood cell. Unlike other cancer cells, which spread from one site, leukemia is a widespread disorder of the marrow and other tissues involved in the blood-forming process.

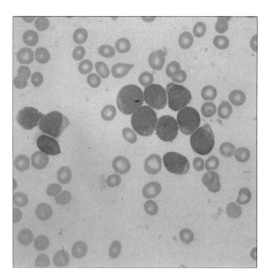

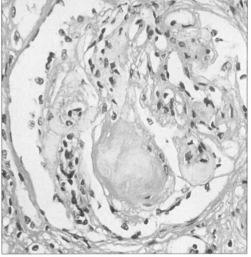

Kidney tissue slice
The slide at left shows a single filtering unit (glomerulus) in a slice of kidney tissue from a person with diabetes. The diabetes has caused some disruption to the structure of the glomerulus (which would normally show more organization). This abnormality would be obvious to a pathologist examining the slide.

Examining tissue
The light microscope provides direct visual evidence of disease in body tissue. The model shown at right is linked to a video monitor, on which a specimen of heart tissue from an AIDS patient is visible.

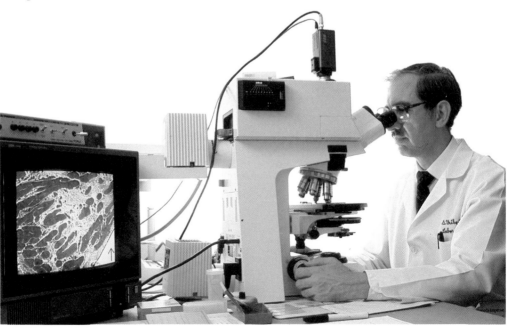

CHAPTER SIX

PRENATAL DIAGNOSIS

INTRODUCTION

SCREENING THE UNBORN BABY

A PREGNANT WOMAN today is offered a bewildering variety of tests. Some of them, such as urine tests, blood pressure checks, and certain blood tests, are primarily concerned with her health, and thus indirectly with the health of her unborn child. Some tests involve checking directly on the baby's health and safety so that any problems – such as a heart defect or awkwardly positioned placenta – can be evaluated and the best timing and method of delivery can be planned. Certain fetal abnormalities can be corrected surgically while the baby is still in the uterus. Doctors may also recommend to prospective parents that one or more tests be performed to determine whether the baby has a severe, untreatable handicap or a serious genetic defect. These tests can be divided into three groups – tests for anatomical abnormalities, such

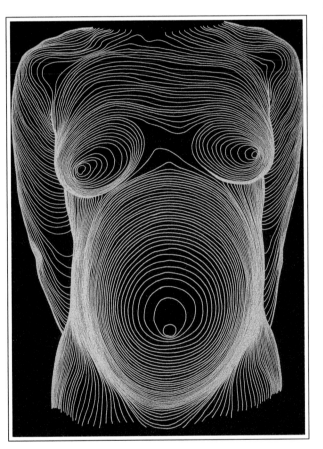

as spina bifida; tests for genetic disorders, such as cystic fibrosis or muscular dystrophy; and tests for chromosome abnormalities, such as Down's syndrome.

This chapter reviews the different techniques used in prenatal diagnosis, which include ultrasound scanning, amniocentesis, and the more recently introduced technique of chorionic villus sampling. It also explains the reasons for having (or

being offered) such tests, the abnormalities these tests can detect, and the circumstances in which there is an increased risk of the baby being affected by an abnormality. These circumstances include relatively advanced maternal age or a family history of a genetic or chromosome disorder. Understanding the risks and benefits of prenatal procedures, and why your doctor may recommend certain tests, helps parents-to-be make informed decisions about which tests they would like to have performed, and so helps them become more involved in the management of the pregnancy. Many parents today choose to be active participants rather than passive onlookers. The doctors involved in your prenatal care can discuss any questions or concerns you may have about prenatal testing in relation to your pregnancy. But within this framework, it is ultimately your choice to approve or refuse a procedure such as ultrasound scanning or amniocentesis. One important point to remember is that there is no single test that can check for everything. Only what is looked for can be found. A negative (good) result for a particular test does not ensure a perfect baby; it indicates only that the baby does not appear to have the condition for which it was tested.

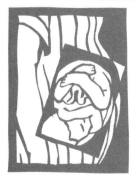

SCREENING THE UNBORN BABY

MANY DIFFERENT TECHNIQUES are available for obtaining images, measurements, and tissue samples of the fetus in the uterus to help diagnose a fetal abnormality. Your doctor may recommend that you undergo some of the procedures discussed here in the course of checking on your health and that of your baby.

The principal techniques used in prenatal diagnosis are blood tests for the mother, ultrasound scanning, amniocentesis, chorionic villus sampling, and fetal blood sampling.

THE MOTHER'S BLOOD

A blood test is performed when pregnancy is confirmed. The blood is checked for signs of anemia, blood type is determined, and tests are performed to rule out conditions that might seriously affect the baby, such as syphilis, HIV (the AIDS virus) infection, and rubella (or lack of immunity to rubella). In women with the Rhesus (Rh)-negative blood group, checkups continue throughout pregnancy for Rh antibodies that might attack the baby's blood.

Another blood sample is usually taken at around 16 weeks and tested for alpha-

Ultrasound scanning
Ultrasound scanning is used as a diagnostic tool to date the pregnancy and to check on its progress. Remarkably clear images of the fetus can be obtained. Ultrasound is also used as an aid to many other prenatal diagnostic tests.

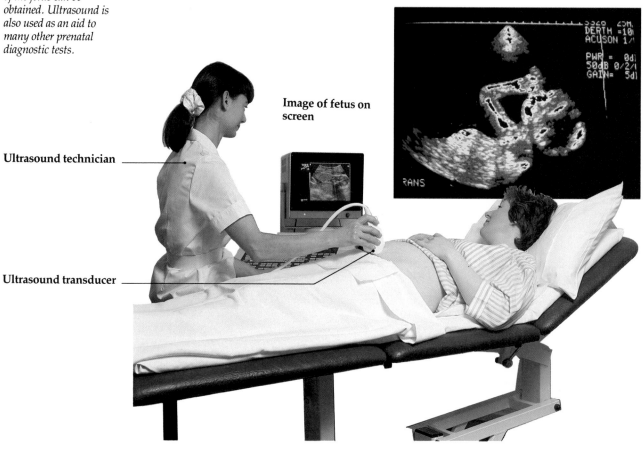

Image of fetus on screen

Ultrasound technician

Ultrasound transducer

fetoprotein to see if the baby is at risk of developing certain abnormalities.

If any of the blood relatives of either parent has had any genetic or chromosomal disorder (or if any of these relatives has had a child who died in infancy for unknown reasons), it is considered that such a disorder may run in the family. Blood samples for some types of genetic disorders can be taken from the parents before or during pregnancy to check on their genetic status.

ULTRASOUND SCANNING

Ultrasound scanning is a method of obtaining an image of the fetus and placenta. It is done by sending short pulses of ultrasonic waves, which can neither be felt nor heard, through the mother's abdomen. The waves produce a picture of structures that are in their path, a bit like sonar (see page 60). Ultrasound scanning is considered risk-free.

What does it show?

In early pregnancy, ultrasound can be used to make sure that the fetus is alive, to date the pregnancy, to check on the location of the placenta, and to determine the number of babies. Later on in pregnancy, ultrasound can be used to check on the position of the baby, on its rate of growth, and on its well-being, as well as to diagnose many anatomical abnormalities in the baby. In a normal pregnancy, many doctors recommend one ultrasound scan at about the fourth month, when provisions can be made for high-risk pregnancy management if necessary. Ultrasound scans may be done more frequently if there is any bleeding from the uterus or if the growth or position of the baby seems abnormal.

Ultrasound is also used as an aid to most of the other diagnostic tests described in this chapter. For example, it is performed both before and throughout amniocentesis (see page 125). Ultrasound enables the doctor to locate the

DOWN'S SYNDROME

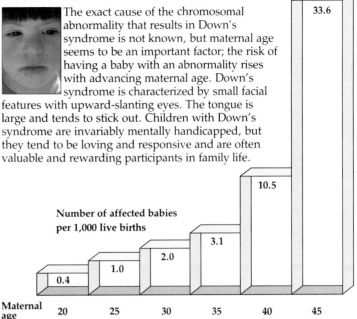

The exact cause of the chromosomal abnormality that results in Down's syndrome is not known, but maternal age seems to be an important factor; the risk of having a baby with an abnormality rises with advancing maternal age. Down's syndrome is characterized by small facial features with upward-slanting eyes. The tongue is large and tends to stick out. Children with Down's syndrome are invariably mentally handicapped, but they tend to be loving and responsive and are often valuable and rewarding participants in family life.

Number of affected babies
per 1,000 live births

Maternal age	20	25	30	35	40	45
	0.4	1.0	2.0	3.1	10.5	33.6

placenta, baby, and amniotic sac, and to see exactly what he or she is doing.

If you have a scan in early pregnancy, you are instructed not to pass urine and, if necessary, to drink several glasses of water beforehand to ensure that you have a full bladder, which acts as a cushion for the uterus, making it more clearly visible on the scan.

FETAL BLOOD SAMPLING

Fetal blood sampling is a test done in rare instances when suitable specimens cannot be obtained by amniocentesis or chorionic villus sampling (see pages 125 and 126). When it is done during pregnancy to check for abnormalities or disease caused by Rh incompatibility, the blood is taken from the umbilical cord near the point where it connects with the placenta. An ultrasound scan is done before and throughout the procedure. The mother is given a local anesthetic and the needle is inserted through her abdominal wall. The results are usually known within a few days. The chance of this procedure causing a miscarriage is about two in 100.

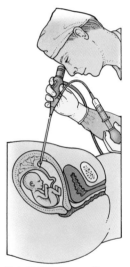

Fetal blood sampling
This procedure is sometimes used during pregnancy to check for abnormalities caused by Rh incompatibility, serious chromosome disorders, or blood disorders. The blood is taken from the umbilical cord near the point where it connects with the placenta.

SCREENING FOR SEVERE ABNORMALITIES

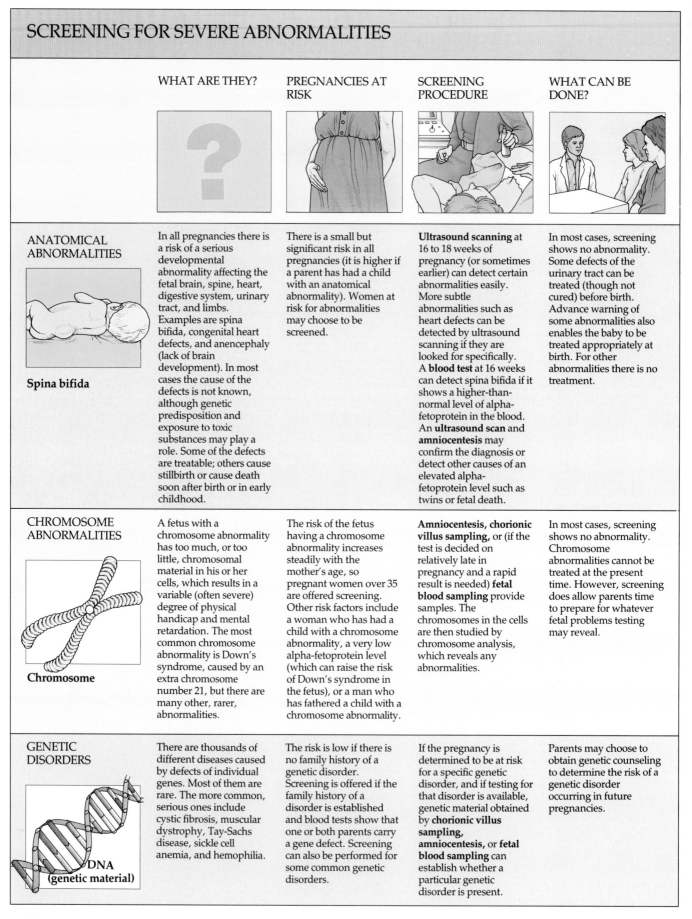

	WHAT ARE THEY?	PREGNANCIES AT RISK	SCREENING PROCEDURE	WHAT CAN BE DONE?
ANATOMICAL ABNORMALITIES **Spina bifida**	In all pregnancies there is a risk of a serious developmental abnormality affecting the fetal brain, spine, heart, digestive system, urinary tract, and limbs. Examples are spina bifida, congenital heart defects, and anencephaly (lack of brain development). In most cases the cause of the defects is not known, although genetic predisposition and exposure to toxic substances may play a role. Some of the defects are treatable; others cause stillbirth or cause death soon after birth or in early childhood.	There is a small but significant risk in all pregnancies (it is higher if a parent has had a child with an anatomical abnormality). Women at risk for abnormalities may choose to be screened.	**Ultrasound scanning** at 16 to 18 weeks of pregnancy (or sometimes earlier) can detect certain abnormalities easily. More subtle abnormalities such as heart defects can be detected by ultrasound scanning if they are looked for specifically. A **blood test** at 16 weeks can detect spina bifida if it shows a higher-than-normal level of alpha-fetoprotein in the blood. An **ultrasound scan** and **amniocentesis** may confirm the diagnosis or detect other causes of an elevated alpha-fetoprotein level such as twins or fetal death.	In most cases, screening shows no abnormality. Some defects of the urinary tract can be treated (though not cured) before birth. Advance warning of some abnormalities also enables the baby to be treated appropriately at birth. For other abnormalities there is no treatment.
CHROMOSOME ABNORMALITIES **Chromosome**	A fetus with a chromosome abnormality has too much, or too little, chromosomal material in his or her cells, which results in a variable (often severe) degree of physical handicap and mental retardation. The most common chromosome abnormality is Down's syndrome, caused by an extra chromosome number 21, but there are many other, rarer, abnormalities.	The risk of the fetus having a chromosome abnormality increases steadily with the mother's age, so pregnant women over 35 are offered screening. Other risk factors include a woman who has had a child with a chromosome abnormality, a very low alpha-fetoprotein level (which can raise the risk of Down's syndrome in the fetus), or a man who has fathered a child with a chromosome abnormality.	**Amniocentesis, chorionic villus sampling,** or (if the test is decided on relatively late in pregnancy and a rapid result is needed) **fetal blood sampling** provide samples. The chromosomes in the cells are then studied by chromosome analysis, which reveals any abnormalities.	In most cases, screening shows no abnormality. Chromosome abnormalities cannot be treated at the present time. However, screening does allow parents time to prepare for whatever fetal problems testing may reveal.
GENETIC DISORDERS **DNA (genetic material)**	There are thousands of different diseases caused by defects of individual genes. Most of them are rare. The more common, serious ones include cystic fibrosis, muscular dystrophy, Tay-Sachs disease, sickle cell anemia, and hemophilia.	The risk is low if there is no family history of a genetic disorder. Screening is offered if the family history of a disorder is established and blood tests show that one or both parents carry a gene defect. Screening can also be performed for some common genetic disorders.	If the pregnancy is determined to be at risk for a specific genetic disorder, and if testing for that disorder is available, genetic material obtained by **chorionic villus sampling, amniocentesis,** or **fetal blood sampling** can establish whether a particular genetic disorder is present.	Parents may choose to obtain genetic counseling to determine the risk of a genetic disorder occurring in future pregnancies.

AMNIOCENTESIS

Amniocentesis is a procedure that consists of drawing some fluid from the pregnant woman's uterus via a fine needle. The fluid is then studied in a variety of ways to look for fetal abnormalities. Amniocentesis is usually done at about 16 weeks of pregnancy, though new research indicates that it may be possible to perform it as early as 10 weeks.

Does it hurt?
Amniocentesis is quick and simple. Some doctors deaden the woman's skin with a local anesthetic, but many do not because the procedure causes only minimal discomfort. After the test, the woman is advised to rest for the remainder of the day.

How is it done?
After locating the amniotic sac with the help of ultrasound, the doctor inserts the needle into the woman's abdomen and uterus and draws off a small amount of amniotic fluid. The length of time it takes to receive the test results varies. Chromosome analysis takes between 2 and 4 weeks. Some types of genetic studies can be quicker; the alpha-fetoprotein test takes a matter of days.

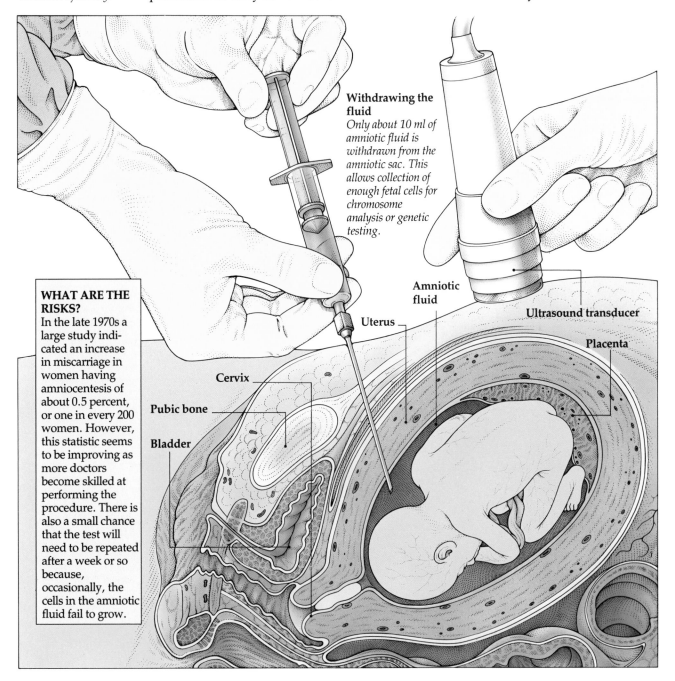

Withdrawing the fluid
Only about 10 ml of amniotic fluid is withdrawn from the amniotic sac. This allows collection of enough fetal cells for chromosome analysis or genetic testing.

WHAT ARE THE RISKS?
In the late 1970s a large study indicated an increase in miscarriage in women having amniocentesis of about 0.5 percent, or one in every 200 women. However, this statistic seems to be improving as more doctors become skilled at performing the procedure. There is also a small chance that the test will need to be repeated after a week or so because, occasionally, the cells in the amniotic fluid fail to grow.

Amniotic fluid

Ultrasound transducer

Placenta

Uterus

Cervix

Pubic bone

Bladder

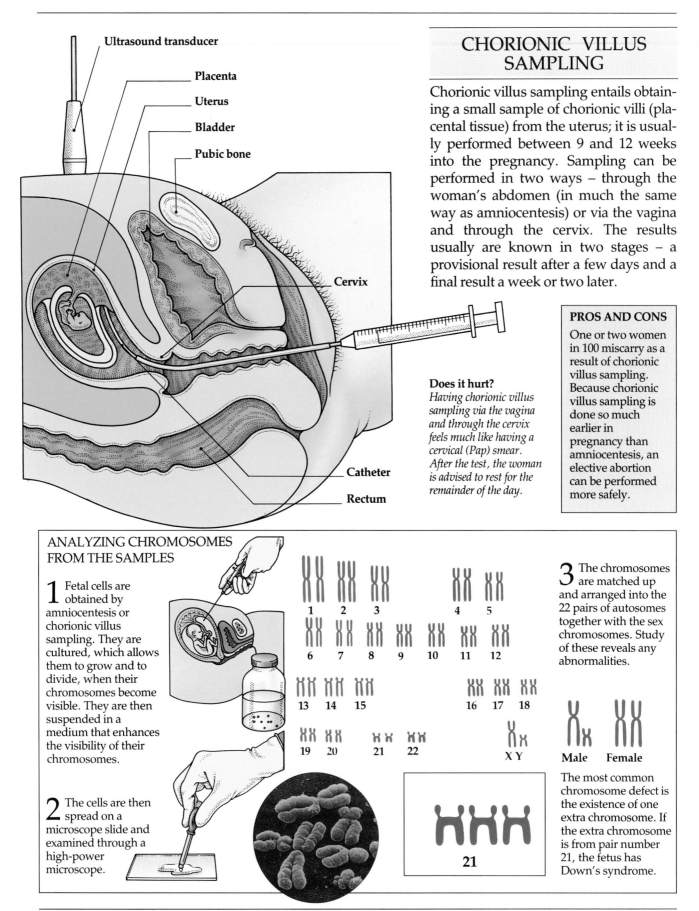

Ultrasound transducer

Placenta

Uterus

Bladder

Pubic bone

Cervix

Catheter

Rectum

CHORIONIC VILLUS SAMPLING

Chorionic villus sampling entails obtaining a small sample of chorionic villi (placental tissue) from the uterus; it is usually performed between 9 and 12 weeks into the pregnancy. Sampling can be performed in two ways – through the woman's abdomen (in much the same way as amniocentesis) or via the vagina and through the cervix. The results usually are known in two stages – a provisional result after a few days and a final result a week or two later.

PROS AND CONS

One or two women in 100 miscarry as a result of chorionic villus sampling. Because chorionic villus sampling is done so much earlier in pregnancy than amniocentesis, an elective abortion can be performed more safely.

Does it hurt?
Having chorionic villus sampling via the vagina and through the cervix feels much like having a cervical (Pap) smear. After the test, the woman is advised to rest for the remainder of the day.

ANALYZING CHROMOSOMES FROM THE SAMPLES

1 Fetal cells are obtained by amniocentesis or chorionic villus sampling. They are cultured, which allows them to grow and to divide, when their chromosomes become visible. They are then suspended in a medium that enhances the visibility of their chromosomes.

2 The cells are then spread on a microscope slide and examined through a high-power microscope.

1 2 3   4 5

6 7 8 9 10 11 12

13 14 15   16 17 18

19 20 21 22   X Y

3 The chromosomes are matched up and arranged into the 22 pairs of autosomes together with the sex chromosomes. Study of these reveals any abnormalities.

Male   Female

The most common chromosome defect is the existence of one extra chromosome. If the extra chromosome is from pair number 21, the fetus has Down's syndrome.

21

CASE HISTORY
AN ENLARGED BLADDER

Holly is the mother of two healthy girls. When she became pregnant with a much-wanted third child, she and her husband, Brad, felt very confident about the pregnancy. Everything went well during the early part of Holly's pregnancy. However, when she went for an ultrasound scan at 19 weeks, the scan showed that all was not as it should be.

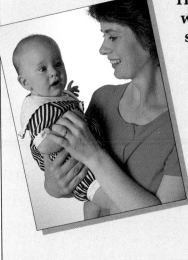

PERSONAL DETAILS
Name Holly Hogan
Age 29
Occupation Part-time receptionist
Family Both Holly and Brad are in good health, and their girls are healthy and growing well. Neither Holly nor Brad is aware of any family history of children born with abnormalities of any kind.

THE CONSULTATION
The ultrasound scan shows that the baby has an enlarged bladder. No other physical abnormality is visible, but the doctor notes that there is an unusually small amount of amniotic fluid in the amniotic sac surrounding the baby in the uterus.

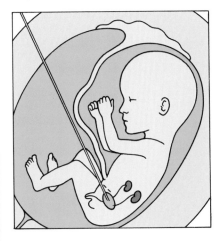

Treating the problem
To treat the baby's urinary blockage, a hollow needle is used to place a tiny drainage catheter in the baby's bladder.

THE DIAGNOSIS
Holly's doctor explains that the most likely cause of the enlarged bladder is a blockage in the urinary system, which is preventing the bladder from emptying.

If the blockage were left untreated, it would eventually lead to kidney damage. Similarly, if the amount of amniotic fluid were not increased, the baby's lungs would fail to mature. The doctor tells Holly and Brad that the baby's life depends on receiving immediate and complicated treatment.

The doctor also explains that urinary tract abnormalities sometimes accompany major chromosome problems, which can also cause mental retardation. Holly and Brad agree that they would like to have the baby's chromosomes tested before deciding on whether or not to begin treatment. Holly is referred to a specialist for fetal blood sampling. Results of amniocentesis take much longer to obtain, so, in situations like Holly's where rapid treatment is needed, fetal blood sampling is often recommended.

FURTHER INVESTIGATION
Holly undergoes fetal blood sampling. The doctor also obtains a sample of urine from the baby's bladder by inserting a needle through Holly's abdominal wall and into its bladder. The urine sample will help determine whether the kidneys are producing normal urine.

THE RESULTS
A week later, Holly and Brad learn that the chromosomes are normal and the kidneys appear to be functioning. They decide to start treatment for the urinary blockage.

THE TREATMENT
Holly is sedated so that she is drowsy but not actually asleep. The skin of her abdomen is anesthetized with a local anesthetic and a hollow needle is inserted through her abdomen and into the baby's bladder. A tiny catheter is then guided through the needle; one end is left in the baby's bladder and the other is left in the amniotic sac. In this way, the bladder is now able to drain.

More ultrasound scans are done in the weeks that follow. For many weeks, the catheter stays in place and functions well. Then, at 36 weeks of pregnancy, an ultrasound scan shows that the catheter has moved out of position in the baby's bladder. The doctor tells Holly and Brad he would like to induce labor.

THE BIRTH
Jonathan is born weighing 5 pounds 7 ounces. He requires an immediate operation to correct the blockage in his urinary tract but, thanks to the catheter, neither his kidneys nor his lungs are damaged.

A-Z OF MEDICAL TESTS

Chapters 2 to 6 of this volume describe many of the most important diagnostic procedures that are regularly performed in the doctor's office, the hospital, and the pathology laboratory. However, because there are so many diagnostic tests available today, many of the more specific tests are not covered in great detail. Described in this section, in alphabetical order, are brief overviews of more than 100 other diagnostic procedures and laboratory tests. Each test is described in terms of its purpose, significance for diagnosing disease, and circumstances in which it is performed. If a test or procedure in which you are interested is not listed in this section, refer to the comprehensive index on pages 142 to 144.

ACID-BASE BALANCE (pH) TEST

The body can function properly only when body fluids are neither too acid nor too alkaline (alkali is another term for a base). To find out if this balance is correct, the concentration of hydrogen ions in the blood is measured. The concentration reflects the acid-base balance because acids release hydrogen ions when dissolved. The terms acid-base balance and pH are closely related. Body fluids with a low pH are too acidic, those with a high pH are too alkaline. The kidneys and the lungs are the two main organs responsible for the maintenance of acid-base balance. They work in precise conjunction to counteract diseases causing an alteration in pH.

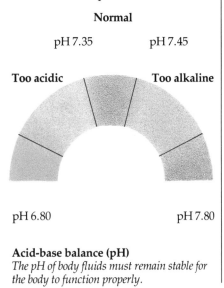

Normal

pH 7.35   pH 7.45

Too acidic   **Too alkaline**

pH 6.80   pH 7.80

Acid-base balance (pH)
The pH of body fluids must remain stable for the body to function properly.

ADRENOCORTICOTROPIC HORMONE MEASUREMENT

Adrenocorticotropic hormone (also called ACTH), which is produced by the pituitary gland, stimulates the outer layer of the adrenal gland to secrete several different hormones. Measurement of the amount of ACTH in the blood can assist in the diagnosis of pituitary and adrenal gland disorders such as Addison's disease and Cushing's syndrome.

ALCOHOL MEASUREMENT

Measuring the body's ethyl alcohol content, which can be done by testing the breath, blood, or urine, is most often related to the legal question of drunk driving. When alcohol is consumed, it reaches a peak in the blood after about 30 minutes; it is then eliminated at the rate of about 1 ounce of ingested alcohol every 3 hours. The blood alcohol test is also an important diagnostic tool when an unconscious person is brought to an emergency facility.

ALDOSTERONE MEASUREMENT

Aldosterone, a hormone produced by the cortex of the adrenal gland, acts on the kidneys to control the amount of salt and water lost in the urine, which in turn affects blood volume and pressure. The test may be performed to investigate the cause of high blood pressure. Raised levels of aldosterone in the blood and urine may indicate a disorder of the kidneys or, in some cases, a tumor of the adrenal glands.

ALPHA-FETOPROTEIN MEASUREMENT

Alpha-fetoprotein (AFP) is a protein usually produced by the fetus. Since it crosses the placenta, it also is found in the mother's blood. Abnormal AFP levels in a pregnant woman's blood at 16 to 18 weeks' gestation may suggest a fetal abnormality, such as spina bifida or Down's syndrome; the AFP level is also abnormal in twin pregnancy. High AFP levels in nonpregnant individuals may occur with some malignant conditions, particularly liver cancer, and with hepatitis.

AMMONIA MEASUREMENT

Ammonia is produced in the body as a waste product from the breakdown of protein. It is normally converted in the liver to urea for excretion by the kidneys. In severe liver disease, such as cirrhosis or acute hepatitis, ammonia can bypass the liver and accumulate in the blood.

ANTIDIURETIC HORMONE MEASUREMENT

Antidiuretic hormone (ADH) is produced by the pituitary gland and acts on the kidneys to reduce the amount of water lost in the urine. This process helps control the body's water balance. Testing the levels of ADH in a person's blood can help in the diagnosis of diabetes insipidus, a disease in which large volumes of urine are produced, usually because of reduced ADH secretion from the pituitary.

ANTINUCLEAR ANTIBODIES TEST

In autoimmune diseases such as systemic lupus erythematosus, the body's immune system may perceive portions of body cell nuclei as foreign and respond by producing antinuclear antibodies (ANAs). The test detects ANAs by examining a blood sample under an ultraviolet microscope. If ANAs are present, they appear to glow. The test may also be used to monitor the effectiveness of therapy.

BICARBONATE MEASUREMENT

Bicarbonate is an important substance for maintaining the blood's acid-base balance (pH). If bicarbonate is lost from the body because of a kidney problem, diarrhea, or other disease, the blood becomes too acid. Bicarbonate is measured in the blood in conjunction with other tests, such as measurement of BLOOD ELECTROLYTES (page 109), and is considered along with the results of measuring arterial BLOOD GASES (page 108) in the evaluation of acid-base balance. The main organs responsible for the maintenance of acid-base balance are the kidneys and the lungs.

BLEEDING TIME

The bleeding time is the time it takes for bleeding to stop after a small puncture is made in the skin. It is normally 3 to 5 minutes. Measurement of the bleeding time can help in the evaluation of bleeding disorders. A prolonged time usually indicates a deficiency of platelets (which help arrest bleeding) in the blood. This can result from ingesting medications that contain aspirin, adverse drug reactions, congenital abnormalities of the platelets, or any other cause of greatly reduced numbers of platelets.

BONE MARROW BIOPSY

All red blood cells, and most white blood cells and platelet-forming cells, are made in the bone marrow, which contains immature forms of these cells. By looking through a microscope at bone marrow cells obtained by aspiration biopsy (page 101), it is possible to diagnose certain diseases, such as leukemia, cancer of the lymphatic system, many forms of anemia, and some other cancers.

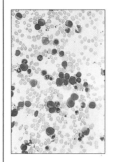

Bone marrow biopsy
In this bone marrow biopsy, taken from a person with megaloblastic anemia, the red blood cells appear faint red and the white blood cells appear purple.

BRONCHOGRAPHY

In this X-ray procedure (done on rare occasions), a substance opaque to X-rays is introduced into the bronchi (the main air passages of the lungs) via a tube passed down the trachea (windpipe). Today, doctors more often examine the bronchi by CT SCANNING (page 48) or BRONCHOSCOPY (page 75).

CALCITONIN MEASUREMENT

Calcitonin, a hormone produced by the thyroid gland, reduces the level of calcium in the blood by slowing the rate at which calcium is lost from bones. A raised level of calcitonin may indicate that a certain type of thyroid cancer is present.

CALCIUM MEASUREMENT

Abnormal calcium levels are common to a variety of diseases. Calcium is usually measured in blood but can be measured in urine, feces, and spinal fluid. Calcium is measured when there are suspected abnormalities of the parathyroid glands (which control the body's calcium needs and use), in vitamin D deficiency, and in bone diseases, especially with kidney failure.

CALORIC TEST

In the caloric test, water at varying temperatures is poured into each of the ear canals, causing stimulation of one of the semicircular canals within the labyrinth. If nystagmus (horizontal jerking movements of the eyes) is absent or lasts for a shorter period of time than normal in one eye, it indicates damage to the labyrinth, part of the inner ear. The test may be used to investigate dizziness or hearing loss.

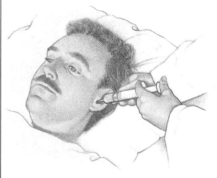

Caloric test
Water is poured into the outer-ear canal and the effect on nystagmus (reflex movement of the eyes) is noted.

CARCINOEMBRYONIC ANTIGEN MEASUREMENT

Carcinoembryonic antigen (CEA) is a protein produced by the fetus in the uterus. Normally, production is halted before birth. Abnormal occurrence of CEA in the blood may be caused by alcoholic hepatitis, obstruction of the bile duct, heavy smoking, and several different types of cancer. The test is not specific for one particular disorder but it may be used to follow and evaluate the effectiveness of therapy for bowel and pancreatic cancers.

CARDIAC BLOOD POOL IMAGING

In this technique, a radioactive substance bound to a blood protein or to red blood cells is injected into the bloodstream and travels to the heart. A special camera is used to detect the radioactivity emitted as blood moves through the heart during each heartbeat. Because more radioactivity is emitted when more blood is present, the difference in blood volume when the heart chambers contract and then relax can be calculated. The test evaluates how efficiently the heart muscle is functioning as a pump.

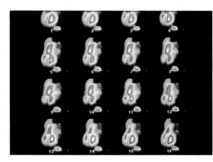

Cardiac blood pool imaging
This series of scans shows one complete heart cycle. The red areas represent blood filling the atria and then the ventricles.

CARDIAC CATHETERIZATION

In this technique, a thin tube is inserted into a vein or artery in the groin or elbow and fed along until its tip enters the right or left side of the heart. A number of tests can then be performed. The blood pressure inside the chambers of the heart can be measured, blood can be drawn off

and its oxygen content measured, and a substance opaque to X-rays can be injected so that the chambers of the heart and the arteries to the heart can be visualized. The efficiency of the heart's contractions can be analyzed using cardiac catheterization; any valve leaks or coronary heart disease can also be detected.

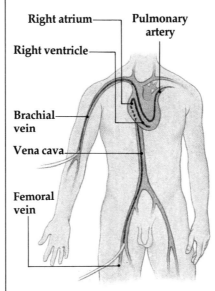

Right-sided cardiac catheterization
A catheter is inserted into the femoral vein or brachial vein and guided until it reaches the right ventricle. The catheter can also be guided farther to enter the pulmonary artery.

CERVICAL PUNCH BIOPSY

This procedure involves the removal, with sharp forceps, of a small tissue specimen from the cervix for further examination under a microscope. It may be carried out in women with suspicious or abnormal cervical (Pap) smears to see if they have any signs of cervical cancer.

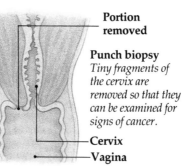

Punch biopsy
Tiny fragments of the cervix are removed so that they can be examined for signs of cancer.

CHOLECYSTOGRAPHY

In this technique the gallbladder and bile ducts are examined by means of X-ray pictures after they have been filled with a substance opaque to X-rays. The substance is taken by mouth, absorbed through the intestinal wall into the bloodstream, and carried to the liver. Several hours later, it is excreted into the bile ducts and gallbladder. Cholecystography can detect gallstones but is rarely done for this purpose. ULTRASOUND SCANNING (page 60) is preferred. However, cholecystography is being used for patients who are candidates for lithotripsy and chemical dissolution of gallstones. This test shows whether the gallbladder functions, and suggests the nature of the stones.

CHOLYLGLYCINE MEASUREMENT

Cholylglycine is a bile acid. Bile is produced by the liver, stored in the gallbladder, and then excreted into the intestine where it helps in the digestion of fats. It is then absorbed back into the liver. In the early stages of any liver disease, the uptake of bile is disrupted, causing an increase in the level of bile acids, such as cholylglycine, in the blood.

CLOTTING FACTOR MEASUREMENT

The blood contains many proteins that are vital to blood clotting. The level of many of these proteins in the blood can be individually measured to ascertain the cause of bleeding disorders as an adjunct to other BLOOD CLOTTING TESTS (page 104).

COLD AGGLUTININS MEASUREMENT

Cold agglutinins are antibodies that cause red blood cells to stick together at low temperatures. Elevated levels of these antibodies in the blood develop during certain infectious diseases, notably some types of pneumonia. Cold agglutinins are therefore measured to confirm certain cases of pneumonia.

COLOR VISION TESTS

These tests are used to assess patients with suspected disease of the retina or with a family history of color vision deficiency. They are also often performed on children. The most common color vision tests use plates made up of a group of dots of related colors (such as reds and pinks) superimposed on backgrounds of another group of colors (such as greens and blues). A person with normal color vision can identify the dot pattern; someone with a color deficiency cannot distinguish between the pattern and the background or misreads the pattern.

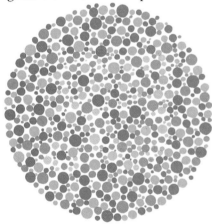

Color vision test
This illustration shows a typical plate used to test color vision. People with color vision deficiency fail to read the number 57.

COMPLEMENT MEASUREMENT

Complement is a group of proteins in the blood that helps destroy foreign cells and remove foreign material. A deficiency of complement increases susceptibility to infection and other diseases. A variety of tests can measure the function of differ-

ent components of complement. They help establish the diagnosis of immune system disorders.

COPPER MEASUREMENT

Copper is a mineral needed in trace amounts. Measurement of its levels in the blood, and sometimes in the urine, is useful in diagnosing hepatolenticular degeneration, in which copper becomes trapped in organs such as the liver, brain, and in the rim of the cornea. A low level of copper indicates hepatolenticular degeneration. Increased levels may occur in conditions such as anemia or liver cirrhosis, during pregnancy, and in a person who is taking contraceptive pills.

CORTISOL MEASUREMENT

Cortisol, a hormone secreted by the outer layer of the adrenal gland, controls the breakdown of proteins, regulates the immune system, and helps maintain correct body water and mineral distribution. Measurement of its blood levels can assist in the diagnosis of hormonal disorders such as Cushing's syndrome (caused by increased cortisol secretion) and Addison's disease (caused by decreased or absent secretion).

C-REACTIVE PROTEINS, BLOOD DETECTION OF

C-reactive proteins may appear in the blood in response to inflammation. They can occur in bacterial and viral infections, rheumatic fever, arthritis, heart attack, and cancer. Detection of C-reactive proteins is not specific for any particular disease, but is an indicator of the presence of an underlying disorder that may require further study.

CREATININE CLEARANCE TEST

Creatinine is a body waste product filtered from the blood by the kid-

neys and excreted in the urine. The creatinine clearance test determines the rate at which blood is filtered by measuring the amount of creatinine in the blood and the amount in a sample of urine collected over a period of 24 hours. This test provides a reliable indicator of how well the kidneys are working.

CYSTOMETRY

This procedure measures the change in pressure in the bladder as it fills, the total bladder capacity, and bladder sensation. A flexible tube is inserted through the urethra into the bladder and the end outside the body is attached to a pressure gauge. The bladder is then filled with a measured volume of water or carbon dioxide and a series of pressure readings are taken. The test provides information about bladder function and can help establish the cause of incontinence.

CYSTOURETHROGRAPHY

A substance opaque to X-rays is introduced through the urethra into the bladder so that the outline of the bladder and urethra will show up in detail on X-rays taken during urination. The test is most commonly performed on young children who have had urinary tract infections to see if the cause is a reflux of urine back up one of the ureters as the bladder empties. Cystourethrography is also performed without X-rays by utilizing a radionuclide substance.

DRUG SCREENING TESTS

These tests are used in emergency departments of hospitals to determine the type and amount of legal or illegal drugs taken in an overdose. They are also used to monitor absorption levels in workers exposed to toxic substances. Levels of medications taken by a patient can also be measured in this way.

ELECTRO-NYSTAGMOGRAPHY

Nystagmus is a reflex movement of the eye that occurs in response to head movement, the introduction of warm and cool water into the ear canals, and certain other stimuli. Electronystagmography detects and quantifies nystagmus by recording electrical changes caused by eye movement via electrodes attached to the skin near the eye. It is quantitative and more comprehensive than the caloric test. Electronystagmography may be performed on people suffering from dizziness, hearing loss, or ringing in the ears. Abnormal or absent nystagmus indicates that the balance mechanisms are not working properly.

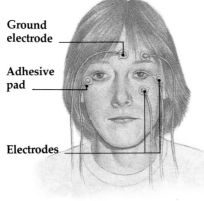

Ground electrode

Adhesive pad

Electrodes

Electronystagmography
Electrodes attached to the skin around the eyes accurately detect nystagmus (reflex eye movement).

ESTROGEN MEASUREMENT

Estrogen is a female sex hormone produced mainly by the ovaries. Estrogen levels in the blood or urine may be measured to establish the cause of infertility, delayed puberty, or menstrual disorders. An abnormally high level may be caused by cirrhosis, a tumor that produces estrogen, or cancer of the testicle. One type of estrogen, estriol, is produced by the placenta and excreted in the mother's urine.

FERRITIN MEASUREMENT

Ferritin is a protein involved in the storage of iron in the body. The amount that appears in the blood is directly proportional, in the absence of other diseases, to the amount of iron stored in the body tissues. Measurement of blood ferritin levels may be carried out to diagnose long-standing iron deficiency, or to help diagnose various disorders that result in increased iron levels, such as liver disease, leukemia, or chronic infection or inflammation.

FIBRINOGEN MEASUREMENT

Fibrinogen is an important component of the blood's clotting system. When a blood vessel is injured, fibrinogen is converted to fibrin, which forms fibrous filaments that plug the damaged vessel. Fibrinogen is measured to determine whether a low level is responsible for abnormal bleeding. Causes of low fibrinogen levels include severe liver disease, cancer of the prostate, pancreas, or lung, a congenital deficiency, or when excessive clotting is taking place in the body, which can occur in disseminated intravascular coagulopathy or chronic bleeding.

FIBRINOLYTIC SPLIT PRODUCTS MEASUREMENT

Fibrinolytic split products (FSPs) are protein fragments that are released into the blood after a clot has formed to seal an injured blood vessel. FSPs prevent the formation of abnormal blood clots, which can clog the circulation. The test is carried out to find out whether a high level of FSPs is the cause of blood failing to clot, resulting in prolonged or excessive bleeding. FSP levels in the blood are also elevated in a syndrome called disseminated intravascular coagulopathy, in which clotting within small blood vessels takes place abnormally throughout the body.

FLUORESCEIN EYE STAIN

Fluorescein is an orange dye that is used to examine the cornea (the front surface of the eye). Drops containing the dye are placed onto the eye, and the eye is examined under ultraviolet light. The fluorescein glows yellow, showing up any irregularities of the cornea, including scratches, ulcers, or areas that have been damaged by infection.

Corneal ulcer

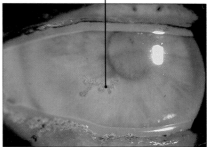

Fluorescein stain
After being stained with the orange dye fluorescein, a corneal ulcer is revealed in bright yellow color under ultraviolet light.

FOLATES MEASUREMENT

Folates, a group of vitamins that includes folic acid, are needed to produce red blood cells in the bone marrow. A deficiency can lead to anemia. These vitamins are found in a variety of foods, particularly in liver and raw vegetables. Because the body is only able to store small amounts of folates, an inadequate intake in the diet soon leads to a deficiency. There is a greater risk of deficiency during pregnancy.

FOLLICLE-STIMULATING HORMONE MEASUREMENT

Follicle-stimulating hormone (FSH) is produced by the pituitary gland and stimulates activity in the gonads (the ovaries in women and the testicles in men). The test is used to investigate infertility in both men and women and menstrual disorders in women. An FSH measurement may also be performed to help in the diagnosis of precocious puberty in children.

GALACTOSEMIA SCREENING TEST

This test is performed on newborn babies to check for the presence of the enzyme that converts galactose (a sugar derived from the milk sugar lactose) into glucose (another type of sugar). A small amount of blood is placed onto specially treated filter paper and examined for signs of fluorescence under ultraviolet light. Normal blood shows fluorescence. Blood deficient in the enzyme does not. If the enzyme is found to be lacking, the baby is fed with special lactose-free milk to prevent a build-up of galactose in the blood, a condition known as galactosemia. If the baby were not fed lactose-free milk, cataracts, liver disease, and mental retardation would develop.

GASTRIC ACID SECRETION TEST

This test is used to determine whether the stomach is secreting gastric acid. Fluid is drawn out of the stomach and sent to the laboratory for analysis. An injection to stimulate the production of gastric acid is then given and the gastric juice is collected again. High levels of acid may indicate the presence of an ulcer or a rare tumor that stimulates acid production. The measurement of gastric acid may also help in the diagnosis of pernicious anemia and stomach disorders.

GASTRIN MEASUREMENT

Gastrin is a hormone produced by the cells in the stomach and, to a lesser extent, by the pancreas in response to eating. Gastrin stimulates the stomach to release acid and the pancreas to produce insulin; it also increases the contraction of the muscles in the wall of the stomach and intestine so that food is propelled through the digestive tract. The test is performed when there are multiple, severe, recurrent stomach and duodenal ulcers. A high level of gastrin indicates the presence of a gastrin-secreting tumor, often located in the pancreas.

GLUCAGON MEASUREMENT

Glucagon is a hormone produced by the pancreas that stimulates the breakdown of glycogen (a carbohydrate stored in the liver and muscles) into glucose (blood sugar). The glucose is carried in the bloodstream and can be used for energy by cells anywhere in the body. Glucagon measurement is performed when hypoglycemia (low blood sugar) is suspected, to monitor diabetes, and to aid in the diagnosis of certain rare tumors of the pancreas.

GLUCOSE-6PD MEASUREMENT

Glucose-6-phosphate dehydrogenase (G6PD) is an enzyme normally found in red blood cells. This test is performed on any person with a family history of G6PD deficiency. If deficiency is confirmed, the person must avoid certain drugs and foods that can precipitate the destruction of large numbers of red blood cells, which can lead to anemia.

GONORRHEA, TESTS FOR

Gonorrhea is a sexually transmitted disease that primarily affects the urethra and genitals. The bacterium *Neisseria gonorrhoeae* is responsible. To test for gonorrhea, Gram's stain is added to a sample of penile or vaginal discharge for viewing under the microscope. If present, the bacteria can be seen inside white blood cells in distinct L-shaped pairs. Culture of the sample confirms the test.

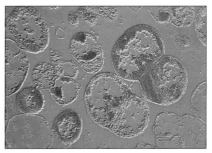

Gonorrhea bacteria
This color-enhanced microscope picture shows Neisseria gonorrhoeae *bacteria.*

GROWTH HORMONE MEASUREMENT

Growth hormone, also known as human growth hormone (HGH), is secreted by the pituitary gland and is essential for normal growth. Measurement of its levels is used in the diagnosis of growth disorders such as pituitary dwarfism and in cases of overproduction of the hormone.

HEPATITIS, TESTS FOR

Viral hepatitis is a serious liver infection caused by any of several viruses. If viral hepatitis is suspected, a blood sample is tested for antibodies to the viruses and sometimes for viral antigens (viruses or portions of the virus). The tests may reveal whether the patient has been exposed to a hepatitis virus, the specific type of virus, the stage of any current infection, and whether the patient is a carrier of hepatitis antigens that could be infectious.

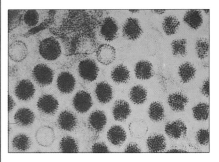

Hepatitis A viruses
This electron microscope picture shows several of the viruses responsible for causing one type of hepatitis.

HETEROPHIL AGGLUTINATION TEST

This test is used to help diagnose infectious mononucleosis. A sample of blood taken from a person suspected of having the disease is mixed with red blood cells from sheep in a test tube. The blood of infected people contains antibodies (proteins produced by the immune system to counter the virus) that cause the sheep cells to clump together. Some other antibodies may also cause clumping, so more specific tests may be needed.

HLA DETERMINATION

HLA stands for human leukocyte antigens – a group of chemical markers present on all cells but most often detected on a person's white blood cells (leukocytes). Determination of a person's individual group of HLAs, his or her tissue type, is needed for an organ transplant operation. A person's HLAs also can have diagnostic significance because certain diseases are strongly associated with particular HLAs. The spinal disorder ankylosing spondylitis rarely occurs except in people with the HLA group HLA-B27.

HUMAN PLACENTAL LACTOGEN MEASUREMENT

Human placental lactogen (HPL) is a hormone produced by the placenta (the organ that links the blood supplies of a pregnant woman and her baby). HPL appears in the blood in about the fifth month of pregnancy, gradually increases until the baby is born, and then disappears.

HYSTEROSALPINGOGRAPHY

This X-ray examination of the uterus and fallopian tubes may be performed to investigate the cause of infertility. A dye opaque to X-rays is passed into the uterus and fallopian tubes through a tube inserted into the cervix (neck of the uterus), and X-ray pictures are taken. The procedure can reveal abnormalities, such as blockage of the tubes or alterations in the shape of the uterus.

IMMUNOGLOBULINS MEASUREMENT

Immunoglobulins are proteins manufactured by the white blood cells to defend the body against disease. The levels of five different types of immunoglobulins can be tested for in a blood sample. Immunoglobulins are measured in cases of obscure infection, in the assessment of disorders of the immune system, and in cases of some malignant tumors in which abnormal immunoglobulin proteins are produced by the tumor cells.

IMPOTENCE TESTS

Also called penile function tests, impotence tests are used to determine whether a man's inability to achieve an erection has a physical cause (such as illness or certain drugs), a psychological cause, or both. These tests may include measurement of blood hormone levels, diabetes screening, nerve conduction studies, studies of penile blood vessels, penile pressure measurements, and measurements of erection while the man is asleep. If it can be shown that erections occur during sleep (a normal occurrence in healthy men), failure to achieve erections when awake is presumed to be psychological in origin. While the man sleeps, electrodes are attached to his head and penis. The electrodes measure levels of sleep and swelling of the penis throughout the night. A portable monitoring device can be used at home. Sensor rings are placed around the penis, and the number, size, and duration of erections are recorded on a counter.

INSULIN MEASUREMENT

Measurement of the amount of insulin in the blood is used to help diagnose diabetes and tumors of the pancreas (which secrete insulin). Blood is tested after the person has fasted for 12 hours. A measured amount of glucose (sugar) is then given and blood insulin is measured every half hour for 3 to 4 hours. Lower-than-normal amounts are found with diabetes and higher-than-normal amounts are found with certain pancreatic tumors.

INTELLIGENCE TESTING

Intelligence tests are performed to assess the mental skills and learning ability of individuals or groups in comparison with the general population. Most of the tests focus on the use of learning, reasoning ability, and memory in solving problems. A common problem in determining the accuracy of results lies in taking sufficient account of the background and environment of the person being tested. For this reason, performance tests that do not rely heavily on verbal ability are often preferred for assessing the general intelligence quotient (IQ).

INTRINSIC FACTOR LEVEL

The intrinsic factor is a protein in the secretions of the stomach that joins with dietary vitamin B_{12} to facilitate its absorption into the bloodstream. Failure of the factor to bond with the vitamin results in defective formation of red blood cells due to vitamin B_{12} deficiency (pernicious anemia). Measuring the levels of intrinsic factor in the blood shows whether vitamin B_{12} is being absorbed correctly.

IRON MEASUREMENT

Iron is essential for the formation of the oxygen-carrying components in blood and muscle. Measuring the amount of iron in the blood is often done to investigate the cause of persistent weakness or tiredness. Low levels of iron are found in anemia, infections, and cancers. In some cases, excessive iron is absorbed and stored in the body, leading to high levels of iron in the blood. One cause of this state is hemochromatosis, an inherited disease.

JEJUNAL BIOPSY

The jejunum is the middle, coiled section of the small intestine. It cannot be entirely examined by endoscopy, so a special intestinal biopsy capsule is used when a sample of tissue is required. First, the person swallows the capsule, which is attached to a thin tube. An X-ray is taken to confirm that the capsule has reached the jejunum, and a syringe attached to the tube is used to suck a tiny section of tissue into the capsule, where the tissue is cut. The capsule is then withdrawn and the sample removed for examination.

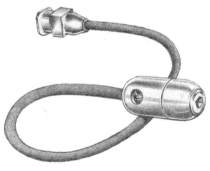

Jejunal biopsy capsule
This small capsule is swallowed and used to take a tissue sample from the jejunum (part of the small intestine).

KETONES MEASUREMENT

Ketones are substances produced when fat is metabolized. Excessive amounts are produced when glucose is not available as a source of energy, forcing the body to use its stores of fat, which occurs in starvation and inadequately treated diabe-

tes mellitus. This test is used to monitor diabetes and some forms of weight reduction.

KIDNEY STONE ANALYSIS

Kidney stones that have been passed in the urine or removed surgically from the kidneys, ureters, or bladder are examined for their chemical constituents. Kidney stone analysis helps determine whether the stones have been caused by infection or by excessive amounts of calcium, oxalate, or uric acid salts.

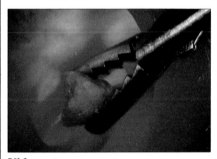

Kidney stone
This kidney stone, shown being removed via an endoscope, will be analyzed in the laboratory.

LACTOSE TOLERANCE TEST

This test is used to detect an inability to digest lactose, a sugar found in milk. Blood sugar levels are measured after the person has fasted for 8 to 12 hours. He or she is then given liquid lactose, and blood sugar is measured again about an hour later. Failure of the blood sugar level to rise indicates that lactose has not been broken down to glucose and galactose, and that there is an intolerance to lactose, often due to a deficiency of the enzyme lactase.

LEAD MEASUREMENT

Lead is a trace element that can produce a toxic reaction when it enters the body in excess. Measuring its levels in the blood or urine can help confirm a diagnosis of lead poisoning suggested by other findings.

LIPASE MEASUREMENT

Lipase is an enzyme secreted by the pancreas, which helps to break down triglycerides (types of fat) so that they can be utilized by the body. Lipase levels in the blood are measured to investigate pancreatic disease. The lipase levels usually parallel those of another enzyme produced by the pancreas (amylase), and the two are sometimes measured at the same time.

LIPIDS MEASUREMENT

Lipids are fatty substances that include triglycerides (the principal component of body fat), phospholipids, and steroids such as cholesterol. Measuring the levels of these lipids in the blood is important in assessing a person's risk of coronary heart disease. Some people have an inherited tendency to high blood levels of one type of lipid.

LIPOPROTEINS MEASUREMENT

Lipoproteins form as the result of lipids (fatty substances in the body) combining with protein molecules. They are classified according to their density, into very low-density lipoproteins (VLDLs), low-density lipoproteins (LDLs), and high-density lipoproteins (HDLs). Lipoproteins are measured to help determine the risk of heart and artery disease. High levels of LDL and low levels of HDL are associated with increased risks of heart and artery disease.

LUTEINIZING HORMONE MEASUREMENT

Luteinizing hormone (LH) is secreted by the pituitary gland and acts on the ovaries to control ovulation and the menstrual cycle. Measurement of the level of LH in the blood is used to assess infertility, to detect ovulation, to evaluate amenorrhea (cessation of periods), and to monitor therapy designed to induce ovulation. For accurate diagnosis, results must be evaluated along with other related hormone tests.

LYMPH NODE BIOPSY

A lymph node biopsy consists of the surgical removal of a small piece of lymphatic tissue for examination under a microscope. The procedure may be done to determine the cause of lymph node enlargement or to confirm the diagnosis of lymphoma (lymphatic system cancer). A piece of tissue may be cultured if an infectious disease is suspected to be causing enlarged lymph nodes.

LYMPHOCYTE TESTS

Lymphocytes are types of white blood cells and are the most important components of the immune system. They fall into two main types, called B cells and T cells. A count of the total number, and of the proportions, of different types of lymphocytes in a blood sample (lymphocyte assays) aids in the diagnosis of various forms of leukemia and immune deficiency disorders. Lymphocyte transformation tests evaluate lymphocyte function – their ability to respond to foreign substances or disease organisms entering the body – and also help in the diagnosis of immune deficiency disorders.

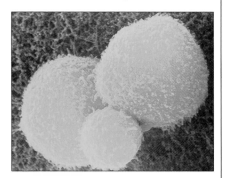

Lymphocyte
This color-enhanced microscope picture shows a T-lymphocyte killer cell attacking two larger cancer cells.

MAGNESIUM MEASUREMENT

Magnesium is one of the most abundant minerals in the body and is found in all cells, but the two largest body stores are in the muscle and bone. Magnesium is active in many biochemical processes. It is important in regulating the body's calcium supply and usage, so measuring its levels in the blood is usually done in conjunction with a calcium test. The test is performed when a person displays signs of magnesium deficiency, such as twitching muscles, irritability, and weakness.

MINNESOTA MULTIPHASIC PERSONALITY INVENTORY

The Minnesota Multiphasic Personality Inventory (MMPI) is a psychological test used to construct a profile of an individual's personality. More than 500 separate statements, such as "I feel people do not like me," are presented to the subject, who is asked to indicate whether he or she agrees, disagrees, or cannot say. The test is used in schools as a counseling aid and in business to screen prospective employees. The accuracy and value of this personality test are not universally accepted by the medical profession.

MYELOGRAPHY

Myelograpy is an X-ray examination in which a substance opaque to X-rays (contrast medium) is injected into the spinal canal so that the spinal cord, spinal nerves, and other tissues within the spinal canal can be seen. The technique has been widely used in the past for diagnosing prolapsed discs ("slipped" discs), tumors in the spinal canal, and nerve injuries. Today, myelography is being replaced by newer, highly accurate, less invasive imaging techniques such as MAGNETIC RESONANCE IMAGING (page 54).

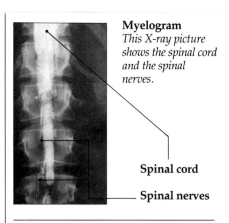

Myelogram
This X-ray picture shows the spinal cord and the spinal nerves.

Spinal cord

Spinal nerves

NERVE CONDUCTION STUDIES

Nerve conduction studies measure the speed at which electrical impulses are carried along a nerve. They are used to aid diagnosis of nerve injuries, inflammation, and degeneration. The nerve being tested is stimulated by an electrode attached to the skin. Another electrode, at a known distance from the first, picks up the electrical impulses that have traveled along the nerve. The speed at which the impulse traveled can then be calculated.

PARATHYROID HORMONE MEASUREMENT

Parathyroid hormone is produced by the parathyroid glands and regulates the concentration of calcium and phosphorus in the blood. Measurement of parathyroid hormone levels is usually done if blood calcium levels are found to be high. This helps identify overactivity of the parathyroid glands.

PHENYLKETONURIA SCREENING TEST

An abnormally high level of the amino acid phenylalanine in the blood indicates that there is a congenital deficiency of the liver enzyme that normally breaks down phenylalanine into other chemicals (a condition called phenylketonuria). The test is performed routinely on a sample of blood taken from the heel of all newborn babies. If the results are positive, the infant is started on a low phenylalanine diet to prevent permanent mental retardation.

PHOSPHATE MEASUREMENT

Phosphates are constituents of bone and play a part in regulating the acid-base balance (pH) in body fluids. Measurement of phosphate levels in the blood and urine may help in the diagnosis of bone, kidney, and hormonal disorders.

PLASMA VOLUME MEASUREMENT

The plasma is the fluid part of blood in which blood cells are suspended. To calculate its volume, a measured dose of a blue dye is injected into a vein; after the dye has spread through the circulation, a blood sample is taken and the amount of dye present is noted. From the degree of dilution, the plasma volume can be calculated. Measuring the plasma volume is sometimes used for investigating dehydration, edema (accumulation of fluid in tissues), malnutrition, and obesity.

PLASMINOGEN MEASUREMENT

Plasminogen is a protein that is able to dissolve blood clots. A deficiency may result in increased clotting and, in some cases, blockage of blood vessels by clots.

PORPHYRINS MEASUREMENT

The porphyrias are a group of rare disorders caused by inborn errors of metabolism in which there is a fault in the biochemical formation of the blood pigment hemoglobin. Porphyrins are chemicals produced in the body during this process. Measuring the levels of porphyrins in a person's urine can help in the diagnosis of porphyrias.

POTASSIUM MEASUREMENT

Potassium helps maintain the balance of fluids within body cells, assists enzyme reactions, and regulates heart muscle action. Deficiency is usually due to a reaction to medication. Excess potassium may be caused by kidney failure, liver disease, or a deficiency of a hormone made by the adrenal gland. It can be measured in the blood, urine, sweat, saliva, and spinal fluid.

PROGESTERONE MEASUREMENT

Progesterone is a hormone produced by the ovaries that helps regulate the menstrual cycle. Measuring the levels of progesterone in the blood can help in assessing ovarian function as part of infertility studies or in evaluating the function of the placenta during pregnancy.

PROLACTIN MEASUREMENT

Prolactin is a hormone secreted by the pituitary gland. Because it is essential for lactation (production and secretion of milk after childbirth), prolactin levels are raised during pregnancy and breast-feeding. The hormone is also secreted by the pituitary gland in males and in nonpregnant females. The test is used to diagnose pituitary disorders, particularly when a woman who has just given birth is unable to breast-feed; when a woman has menstrual problems; during pregnancy when fetal difficulties are suspected; and when tumors of the pituitary gland itself are suspected (these tumors can cause prolactin to be secreted in excessive amounts).

PROTEIN MEASUREMENTS

The main proteins in the blood are albumin and immunoglobulins. Protein is measured in kidney and liver disease, when multiple myeloma (a type of bone marrow cancer) is suspected, and when there are problems with nutrient absorption. The results are usually given as the total protein or as a ratio of albumin to immunoglobulin. Protein can also be measured in the urine; the presence of small amounts of albumin in the urine indicates kidney disease.

PROTHROMBIN TIME

Prothrombin time is a measurement of several blood-clotting factors manufactured in the liver from vitamin K, which is found mainly in fish, liver, and green leafy vegetables. The prothrombin time indicates the level of clotting factors in the blood by measuring the time it takes for a blood sample to start clotting after addition of clotting accelerators. It is primarily used to monitor the effectiveness of treatment with anticoagulant drugs.

PUPILLARY REFLEX TEST

The pupils of the eyes open and close in response to different amounts of light, or when focusing near or far. The pupillary reflex is tested by directing a strong light into the eye and by asking the patient to focus on different distances. It is performed if there is any suspicion of eye, brain, or nerve disease.

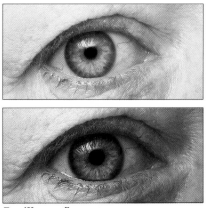

Pupillary reflex test
The pupil normally contracts in strong light and enlarges in weak light.

RADIONUCLIDE THYROID UPTAKE AND SCAN

The main action of the thyroid gland is to convert iodine and other substances into thyroid hormones. Thyroid function can be assessed by measuring the ability of the gland to take in iodine. The test is done by giving an oral dose of radioactive iodine and, after specific intervals, using an external probe to detect the amount of radioactivity in the gland. The scan shows the presence of functioning or nonfunctioning nodules of thyroid tissue.

RED BLOOD CELL INDEXES

The red blood cell indexes are values calculated from the results of other measurements on the red blood cells, such as the red cell count and HEMATOCRIT READINGS (page 103). The indexes provide information about the size of red blood cells and about the weight and concentration of hemoglobin in an average red cell. The red blood cell indexes are of limited benefit in diagnosing the exact nature of anemia.

RED BLOOD CELL SURVIVAL TIME

In hemolytic anemia, red blood cells (whose normal life span is approximately 120 days) are prematurely destroyed in the bloodstream. To aid the evaluation of this condition, a sample of blood is withdrawn, the red cells are labeled with radioactive material, and the blood is then reinjected. A series of blood samples are taken over the next 3 to 4 weeks and the amount of radioactivity measured to give an indication of how many red cells have been destroyed. During this period, the body may also be scanned. Areas of abnormally high radioactivity show the doctor where the greatest numbers of cells are accumulating and being destroyed.

RENIN ACTIVITY MEASUREMENT

Renin is a hormone produced by the kidneys that stimulates the adrenal glands to produce another hormone, aldosterone, which controls blood pressure. The amount of renin in the blood is measured to investigate the cause of high blood pressure, to help determine the type of therapy required, and when adrenal disease is suspected.

RETICULOCYTE COUNT

Reticulocytes are immature red blood cells that can be counted by staining a drop of blood and viewing it under the microscope. A high reticulocyte count indicates that the bone marrow is producing additional amounts of red cells in an attempt to combat anemia or restore blood after profuse bleeding.

RHEUMATOID FACTOR MEASUREMENT

Rheumatoid factor is a type of protein produced by the immune system that is found in the blood of approximately three quarters of people suffering from rheumatoid arthritis. Measurement of rheumatoid factor is used primarily when rheumatoid arthritis is suspected (after a history has been taken and a physical examination performed) to confirm the doctor's diagnosis. Occasionally, the test result is positive in a healthy person.

RORSCHACH TEST

In this psychological test, the subject is asked to interpret a series of inkblots. The Rorschach test is named after its Swiss inventor and has been employed in psychological testing for many years. The diagnostic value of inkblot tests in revealing personality traits is now considered doubtful by many professionals.

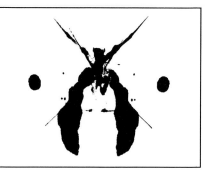

Rorschach test
This is an example of the type of inkblot you are asked to interpret in a Rorschach test.

RUBELLA ANTIBODIES MEASUREMENT

The amount of antibodies to rubella (German measles) in the blood indicates a person's immunity to the disease. If a pregnant woman contracts the disease, especially during the first 3 months of pregnancy, she has a 50 percent chance of giving birth to a child with a congenital defect. All women should be tested before pregnancy. If no rubella antibodies are found, the woman can be vaccinated to bring about immunity.

SCHILLING TEST

This test measures the body's ability to absorb vitamin B_{12} through the intestine. The patient fasts for between 8 and 12 hours and is then given radioactive vitamin B_{12} orally. All urine is collected over the next 24 hours and the amount of radioactive B_{12} in the urine is measured. If little radioactive vitamin B_{12} is excreted, it indicates that the vitamin is not being correctly absorbed.

SCHIRMER'S TEST

This test is performed when a person has dry eyes or when the eyes water constantly. A drop of anesthetic is placed on an eye and a strip of filter paper is placed inside the lower lid. The eyes are kept closed for 5 minutes, the paper is removed, and the amount of fluid is measured.

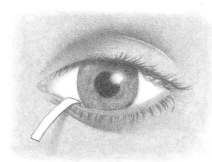

Schirmer's test
Filter paper is inserted into the lower lid as shown, and the amount of moistening is measured.

SEMEN ANALYSIS

Analysis of semen is usually performed to evaluate male fertility, either to discover the cause of infertility or, after a vasectomy, to make sure that the semen no longer contains sperm. Semen analysis may also be used for legal reasons in cases of rape or sexual abuse. To evaluate fertility, a series of semen samples is required. The volume of each sample is measured, the sperm are counted and examined for any abnormalities of shape or motility (ability to move), and a variety of chemical tests are performed.

SEROTONIN MEASUREMENT

Serotonin is one of the chemicals that transmits nerve impulses from one cell to another. The test measures one of the breakdown products of serotonin in the urine. Serotonin may be secreted in excess amounts by certain types of tumors.

SICKLE CELL TEST

Sickle cells are severely deformed red blood cells. As many as one in 700 blacks born in the US has sickle cell anemia, which is diagnosed by the appearance of large numbers of sickle cells in a blood smear viewed under a microscope. Today it is possible to diagnose sickle cell disease in an unborn baby.

SKIN TESTS

Testing the skin's reaction to a range of substances can be a useful aid in the diagnosis of suspected allergy, persistent skin disorders, and certain infections. The skin's reaction to a particular substance may also be evaluated to test the sensitivity of the immune system to that substance. The substance may be introduced to the skin either by injecting the substance just below the skin's surface (an intradermal test) or by soaking a small piece of material in a solution of the substance and then taping it to the skin (a patch test). Many variables can affect the skin's reaction to allergens, which can minimize the value of skin reaction tests in diagnosing allergies.

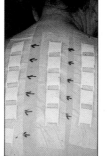

Skin patch test
Suspected allergens are taped to the back (left). Red areas indicate a skin reaction (right).

SODIUM MEASUREMENT

Sodium helps regulate the body's water balance and is necessary for healthy heart, nerve, and muscle function. Measurement of levels of sodium in the blood and urine is done in cases of persistent water retention, to pinpoint the cause of coma, and to diagnose hormonal and kidney disorders.

SPIROMETRY

This procedure is used to help diagnose lung disorders. The person breathes into a spirometer, which records the total volume of exhaled air (forced vital capacity or FVC) and the volume of air exhaled in 1 second (forced expiratory volume in 1 second or FEV$_1$). If the ratio of FEV$_1$ to FVC is less than normal, the person may have an obstructive lung disease, such as asthma, in which the airways are narrowed, resulting in a slower expiration rate. If FVC and FEV$_1$ are reduced about equally, the person is more likely to have a restrictive lung disease with limited lung capacity but normal airways.

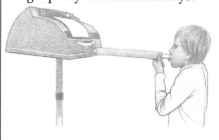

Spirometry
The patient breathes into a spirometer, which records the rate of exhalation and volume of air exhaled.

SWEAT TEST

A raised salt content in sweat is a diagnostic test for the inherited disease cystic fibrosis. Sweating is induced in a patch of skin by contact with the drug pilocarpine. The sweat is collected on filter paper and chemically analyzed.

SYPHILIS, TESTS FOR

Syphilis is a potentially life-threatening sexually transmitted disease that is caused by the spiral-shaped bacterium *Treponema pallidum*. This bacterium is so thin that it is visible only when illuminated by reflected light under a microscope. Syphilis may also be detected by testing the patient's blood for the organism or the antibodies produced against it. False-positive test results for syphilis may occur in patients with immune disorders.

TENSILON TEST

Myasthenia gravis is an immune disorder in which nerve impulses fail to induce normal muscular contraction. If the diagnosis is suspected, a dose of a substance called Tensilon (edrophonium chloride) is given. An immediate increase in muscle strength confirms the diagnosis.

TESTOSTERONE MEASUREMENT

Testosterone is the primary hormone secreted by the testes. It induces puberty in the male and maintains male characteristics. In females, small amounts of testosterone are secreted by the adrenal glands and ovaries. Measurement of testosterone in the blood helps diagnose deficient activity of the testes or ovaries and helps evaluate the cause of male infertility and female hirsutism (excess hair growth on the body) or virilization (masculine physical characteristics in women).

THALLIUM SCANNING

In this type of RADIONUCLIDE SCANNING (page 50), radioactively labeled thallium is injected into a vein and travels to the heart. Areas of the heart that have a normal blood supply and healthy muscle rapidly absorb thallium; any part of the heart in which blood flow is reduced or muscle is damaged takes up less of the radioactive substance. The heart is scanned a few minutes after the injection of thallium to look for any "cold" spots – that is, any areas where there is no radioactivity. The presence of cold spots confirms the existence of muscle damage (due to heart attack) or reduced blood flow (due to coronary heart disease). Thallium scanning is often performed while the patient walks on a treadmill to see whether there is a satisfactory increase in blood flow through the heart during exercise.

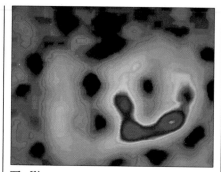

Thallium scan
This color-enhanced scan of the heart shows normal uptake of oxygen (red area).

THYROID HORMONES MEASUREMENT

The measurement of the thyroid hormones triiodothyronine (T_3) and thyroxine (T_4) is performed to assess the function of the thyroid gland, to aid in the diagnosis of thyroid disorders, and to monitor a patient's response to therapy. Most states require routine testing of thyroid hormones in newborn babies. If not treated, abnormally low levels can cause mental retardation and stunted growth.

TORCH SYNDROME TESTS

The acronym TORCH represents a screening panel of blood tests to detect antibodies to toxoplasmosis (a parasitic infection), rubella (German measles), cytomegalovirus, and herpes simplex virus, types I and II. Torch syndrome tests are performed on pregnant women and newborn babies because the five infections have been found to cause blindness, deafness, hepatitis, blood disorders, spleen enlargement, mental retardation, and other defects in the newborn child of an affected woman.

TRANSFERRIN MEASUREMENT

Transferrin is formed in the liver and transports iron around the body. Low levels may indicate inadequate production of transferrin due to liver damage, excessive protein loss from kidney disease, acute or chronic infection, or certain forms of cancer. Elevated levels of transferrin indicate severe iron-deficiency anemia. The level of transferrin in the blood is increased in late pregnancy and during oral contraceptive use.

UREA NITROGEN MEASUREMENT

Urea is produced in the liver and is the primary end product of protein breakdown in the body. It is eliminated by the kidneys into the urine. Normally, there is very little urea in the blood. However, when kidney function is impaired by disease, the level of urea secretion may be decreased even further, causing an increase in urea nitrogen in the blood. The level of urea nitrogen in the blood is also increased in cases of fever or internal bleeding and with certain medications. It is decreased in liver disease and with increased activity of the pituitary gland.

URIC ACID MEASUREMENT

Measurement of the amount of uric acid, a waste product of the body, either in the blood or the urine, is used primarily to help diagnose gout. The test may also be performed to aid in the evaluation of leukemia, toxemia of pregnancy (a condition that can lead to premature labor), and severe kidney damage.

UROBILINOGEN MEASUREMENT

Urobilinogen comes from bilirubin, a yellow pigment formed from the breakdown of red blood cells that is normally excreted by the liver in bile. The urine usually contains small amounts of urobilinogen but, in certain conditions, the level increases. The test is used to help diagnose hemolytic anemia (in which red cells are destroyed at a faster-than-normal rate) and liver damage.

VENOGRAPHY

Venography is an X-ray procedure in which a substance opaque to X-rays is injected into the veins so that they can be examined on X-ray film. It is used to detect abnormalities of the veins themselves, such as narrowing or blockage due to blood clots, tumors, or vascular disease. The veins most commonly examined are those in the leg. Doppler ultrasound scanning of the veins can reveal clots and narrowing without the risk of injecting dye.

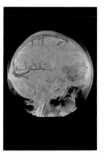

Venogram
This color-enhanced X-ray image shows the network of veins within the skull.

VISUAL ACUITY AND REFRACTION TESTS

To test visual acuity, the patient attempts to read a Snellen's chart, which consists of rows of standard letters of decreasing size. Refraction tests are usually performed using a retinoscope, which projects a beam of light into the person's eyes and allows observation of the light reflected back through the pupil from the retina. The beam is moved in various directions across the pupil while different lenses are placed in front of the eyes to see which will neutralize the movement of light.

VISUAL FIELD TEST

The fields of vision are checked for defects when disease of the retina or optic nerve is suspected. The person looks inside a large, white, hollow hemispherical bowl, fixing his or her gaze on a central target. The doctor causes small, bright spots of light to appear in the bowl and the person presses a button whenever a light is seen. Certain diseases lead to characteristic patterns of visual field loss.

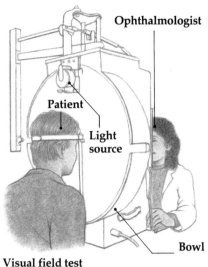

Visual field test
With one eye covered, the patient stares straight ahead into a white bowl while lights are shined onto it.

VITAMINS MEASUREMENT

Deficiencies of certain vitamins can have a variety of damaging effects. Deficiency of vitamin B_{12} can lead to anemia and deficiency of vitamin A can lead to night blindness. Doses of vitamins that exceed the recommended daily allowance can also be harmful. A variety of sensitive chemical tests can help diagnose both deficiency and toxicity. However, too often these tests are done unnecessarily.

WESTERN BLOT TEST

After performing the initial blood test for human immunodeficiency virus (HIV) infection (the AIDS virus) by ELISA (see page 112), the Western blot test is carried out for confirmation. This involves testing for a reaction between HIV antibodies in the patient's serum and actual components of HIV that have been separated out on an absorbent sheet. It is more reliable than ELISA but is technically more difficult.

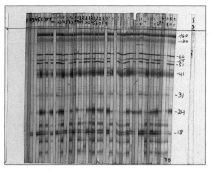

Western blot test
This procedure tests for the AIDS virus. Dark bands at certain positions on the test strips indicate a positive result.

WOOD'S LIGHT EXAMINATION

Wood's light is ultraviolet light from a mercury vapor source; it is used in the diagnosis of skin conditions. Certain fungal infections of the scalp glow green (show fluorescence) under the light. Porphyria, a disorder in which there is a fault in the formation of the blood pigment hemoglobin, glows a coral red.

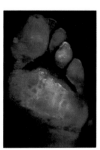

Wood's light examination
The red area on this foot indicates that the person has porphyria.

XYLOSE TOLERANCE TEST

Xylose is a sugar that healthy people absorb from the intestine and excrete unchanged in the urine. Measuring the proportion of a dose (given by mouth) that is excreted in the person's urine helps the doctor test the patient's intestinal function.

ZINC MEASUREMENT

Tiny amounts of zinc are needed to prevent developmental abnormalities, such as growth retardation. Low levels may occur in alcoholism, during pregnancy, after a heart attack or surgery, and in liver disease, cancer, and prostate problems.

INDEX

Page numbers in *italics* refer to illustrations and captions.

Photograph sources:
Science Photo Library **2** (top left); **2** (bottom left); **11** (bottom); **12** (chest X-ray and endoscopist); **37**; **38**; **39**; **42** (top left); **42** (bottom left); **42** (center left); **42** (top right); **42** (center right); **43** (top left); **43** (center left); **43** (top right); **43** (center right); **45**; **46** (left); **46** (right); **47**; **48**; **49**; **50** (right); **51** (top); **52** (top left); **53** (bottom); **57**; **60**; **64** (bottom); **67**; **69** (bottom center) **69** (bottom left); **69** (center right); **69** (bottom right); **70** (bottom); **71** (center right); **74** (top right); **74** (bottom right); **75** (center right); **75** (bottom right); **77** (top right); **77** (inset top right); **80** (bottom right); **82** (bottom right); **85** (bottom inset); **86** (center right); **87**; **96**; **97** (bottom right); **98** (bottom left); **98** (bottom right); **100** (top center); **102** (center right); **102** (bottom right); **102** (bottom left); **103** (bottom right); **104** (top right); **104** (center left); **106** (bottom left); **107** (bottom right); **108**; **109**; **112**; **115** (top); **115** (bottom); **118** (top left); **118** (bottom left); **119** (center); **119** (bottom); **121**; **123** (top center); **126** (bottom); **129**; **130**; **133** (top right); **135** (center); **136** (bottom left); **137** (top and bottom); **140**; **141** (left); **141** (top right)
Dr L.A. Berger **62** (bottom)
Biophoto Associates **103** (top right); **104** (center); **104** (top left); **116** (bottom left)
Daily Telegraph Colour Library **114** (bottom left)

Institute of Dermatology **139** (center left); **139** (center right); **141** (center right)
Middlesex Hospital, Photography and Illustration Centre **86** (normal EEG trace); **86** (petit mal trace)
Moorfields Eye Hospital **132**
National Medical Slide Bank, UK **34** (bottom); **41** (bottom left); **82** (bottom left); **86** (grand mal trace); **99** (bottom right); **100** (bottom left); **101**; **114** (top); **119** (top); **136** (top right)
Network Photographics **15** (crowd background)
Olympus KeyMed **71** (center left); **72** (center right); **73** (inset); **76** (top right); **76** (bottom left); **77** (center right)
Pictor International **2** (center); **7**; **9**; **10**; **12** (test tubes); **12** (microscopist); **13** (ECG recording); **14** (top); **93**
Quantum Medical Systems **65** (left); **65** (right)
Queen Elizabeth Military Hospital, Eye department, Woolwich **81** (top left); **81** (top right); **81** (angiogram sequence)
Barry Richards **86** (top right)
Dr Norbert Roosen **11** (top); **11** (inset top); **51** (bottom)
Dr K.F.R. Schiller, St Peter's Hospital **72** (bottom right); **75** (top)
Siemens, Erlangen **50** (left); **52** (right)
Howard Sochurek **55** (top); **58** (bottom); **59**; **62** (top); **122** (center right)
Dr Paul Sweny **61** (top right); **63** (bottom)
Tony Stone Worldwide **23**; **27**; and **front cover**

C. James Webb **105** (bottom right); **114** (bottom right); **116** (top left); **116** (center left); **117** (top right); **117** (top center); **117** (bottom right); **117** (bottom center); **118** (center); **133** (bottom right)
Dr Robert Youngson **13** (eye examination); **34** (top); **78** (left); **78** (right); **79**; **80** (top left); **80** (top right)

Commissioned photography:
Stephan Oliver
Susanna Price

Illustrators:
David Ashby
Russell Barnet
Karen Cochrane
Andrew Green
David Fathers
Tony Graham
Trevor Hill
Lindum Artists.

Janos Marffy
Coral Mula
Lynda Payne
Howard Pemberton
Lydia Umney
John Woodcock

Charts:
Technical Art Services

Airbrushing:
Roy Flooks
Trevor Hill
Janos Marffy